KNOW YOUR DRUGS

BOOKS BY VERNON COLEMAN

The Medicine Men (1975)
 Paper Doctors (1976)
Everything You Want To Know About Ageing (1976)
Stress Control (1978)
The Home Pharmacy (1980)
Aspirin or Ambulance (1980)
Face Values (1981) Guilt (1982)
The Good Medicine Guide (1982)
Stress And Your Stomach (1983)
Bodypower (1983)
An A to Z Of Women's Problems (1984)
Bodysense (1984)
Taking Care Of Your Skin (1984)
Life Without Tranquillisers (1985)
High Blood Pressure (1985)
Diabetes (1985)
Arthritis (1985)
Eczema and Dermatitis (1985)
The Story Of Medicine (1985)
Natural Pain Control (1986)
Mindpower (1986)
Addicts and Addictions (1986)
Dr Vernon Coleman's Guide To Alternative Medicine (1988)
Stress Management Techniques (1988)
Overcoming Stress (1988)
Know Yourself (1988)
The Health Scandal (1988)
The 20 Minute Health Check (1989)
Sex For Everyone (1989)
Mind Over Body (1989)
Eat Green Lose Weight (1990)
Toxic Stress (1991)
Why Animal Experiments Must Stop (1991)
The Drugs Myth (1992)
Why Doctors Do More Harm Than Good (1993)
Stress and Relaxation (1993)
Complete Guide to Sex (1993)
How to Conquer Backache (1993)
How to Conquer Arthritis (1993)
Betrayal of Trust (1994)
Know Your Drugs (1994)
Food for Thought (1994)

The Traditional Home Doctor (1994)
I Hope Your Penis Shrivels Up (1994)
People Watching (1995)
Relief from IBS (1995)
The Parent's Handbook (1995)
Oral Sex: Bad Taste And Hard To Swallow (1995)
Why Is Pubic Hair Curly? (1995)
Men in Dresses (1996)
Power over Cancer (1996)
Crossdressing (1996)
How To Get The Best Out Of Prescription Drugs (1996)
How To Get The Best Out Of Alternative Medicine (1996)
How to Stop Your Doctor Killing You (1996)
How to Overcome Toxic Stress (1996)
Fighting For Animals (1996)
Alice and Other Friends (1996)
Dr Vernon Coleman's Fast Action Health Secrets (1997)

novels
The Village Cricket Tour (1990)
The Bilbury Chronicles (1992)
Bilbury Grange (1993)
Mrs Caldicot's Cabbage War (1993)
The Man Who Inherited a Golf Course (1993)
Bilbury Revels (1994)
Deadline (1994)
Bilbury Country (1996)

short stories
Bilbury Pie (1995)

on cricket
Thomas Winsden's Cricketing Almanack (1983)
Diary Of A Cricket Lover (1984)

as Edward Vernon
Practice Makes Perfect (1977)
Practise What You Preach (1978)
Getting Into Practice (1979)
Aphrodisiacs - An Owners Manual (1983)
Aphrodisiacs - An Owners Manual (Turbo Edition) (1984)

The Complete Guide To Life (1984)

as Marc Charbonnier
Tunnel (novel 1980)

with Dr Alan C Turin
No More Headaches (1981)

with Alice
Alice's Diary (1989)
Alice's Adventures (1992)

Know Your Drugs

Vernon Coleman

EUROPEAN MEDICAL JOURNAL

European Medical Journal, Publishing House, Trinity Place,
Barnstaple, Devon EX32 9HJ, England

ISBN 1 898947 54 6

Printed and bound in England by J W Arrowsmith, Bristol

Warning

This book is not intended as an alternative to personal, professional medical advice. The reader should consult a physician in all mat-ters relating to health, and particularly in respect of any symptoms which may require diagnosis or medical attention. While the ad-vice and information in this book are believed to be accurate at the time of going to press, neither the author nor the publisher can ac-cept any legal responsibility or liability for any errors or omissions that may be made.

PREFACE

We have become pill poppers – addicted to prescription drugs on a massive scale. On any day you care to choose roughly half the population will be taking a drug of some kind.

Sometimes drugs save lives.

But prescription drugs can also be dangerous. Four out of every ten patients who take prescription drugs suffer nasty – sometimes potentially deadly – side-effects. One in six patients in hospital are there because they have been made ill by the treatment their doctor has given them!

The secret to using drugs safely is to know *what* you are taking – and *why*. And to be aware of any possible side-effects.

Keep *Know Your Drugs* handy and refer to it whenever you need to take a prescription drug.

Vernon Coleman, 1997

PART ONE

ESSENTIAL TIPS FOR PATIENTS
TAKING
PRESCRIPTION DRUGS

HOW TO READ A PRESCRIPTION

When writing out a prescription many doctors still use abbreviations derived from a rough-and-ready version of Latin. The abbreviations are used to give instructions to the pharmacist who will turn the prescription into a bottle of pills. Some of the commonest abbreviations – and their meanings are given below.

If you are confused or uncertain about instructions, or if the instructions on the label don't seem to match the instructions on the prescription, you should check with your doctor immediately – before starting treatment.

ABBREVIATION	LATIN	ENGLISH
aa	ana	of each
ac	ante cibum	before meals
ad lib	ad libitum	freely
alt die	alt diebus	alternate days
alt noct	alt noctibus	alternate nights
aqua calida	aqua calida	hot water
bal	balneum	bath
bd	bis in die	twice a day
bid	bis in die	twice a day
c	cum	with
cat	cataplasma	a poultice
cc	cum	with
cm	cras mane	tomorrow morning
cn	cras nocte	tomorrow evening
dol urg	dolore urgente	when the pain is severe
eq	equalis	equal
ex aq	ex aqua	in water
ext	extractum	extract
f	fiat	let it be made
flav	flavus	yellow
fol	folium	leaf
fs	semi	half
ft	fiat	let it be made
gutt	guttae	drops
haust	haustus	draught
hn	hac nocte	tonight

hor decub	hora decubitus	at bedtime
hs	hora somni	at bedtime
m	misce	mix
m et sign	misce et signa	mix and label
m ft mist	misce fiat mistura	mix and let a mixture be made
md	more dicto	as directed
mdu	more dicto utendus	to be used as directed
mist	mistura	mixture
mit	mitte	send
om	omni mane	every morning
on	omni nocte	every evening
paa	parti effecti applicandus	to be applied to the affected part
p oc	pro oculis	for the eyes
prn	pro re nata	when needed
pulv	pulvis	powder
qd	quater in die	four times a day
qh	quatis horis	four hourly
qid	quater in die	four times a day
qq	quaque	every
qqh	quarta quaque hora	every fourth hour
qs	quantum sufficiat	as much as is sufficient
r	recipe	take thou
rep	repetatur	let it be repeated
rep dos	repetatur dosis	let the dose be repeated
si dol urg	si dolor urgeat	if the pain is severe
sig	signetur	let it be labelled
sos	si opus sit	if necessary
ss	semi	half
stat	statim	immediately
syr	syrupus	syrup
td	ter in die	three times a day
tds	ter die sumendum	three times a day
tert qq hora	tertia quaque hora	every third hour
tid	ter in die	three times a day
ung	unguentum	ointment
ut dict	ut dictum	as directed

FIFTEEN TIPS FOR ANY PATIENT TAKING A PRESCRIPTION DRUG

1. Always follow any specific instructions that you are given by your doctor. Read the label on your bottle of pills and take notice of what it says!

2. When you're not using them, drugs should be stored in a locked cupboard out of reach of children, in a room where the temperature will be fairly stable. The bathroom is probably the worst room in the house for storing medicines. Your bedroom – which probably has a more stable temperature – is much better.

3. Never take drugs which were prescribed for someone else. Return all unused supplies of drugs to your pharmacist.

4. It is wise to assume that all prescribed drugs can cause drowsiness. You shouldn't drive or operate machinery after taking a drug until you are sure that you are safe.

5. Drugs do not mix well with alcohol. If you want to drink while taking drugs ask your doctor whether or not it will be safe.

6. Do not take non-prescribed medicines while taking prescribed drugs unless your doctor has advised you that it is safe and necessary to do so.

7. Do not stop taking drugs suddenly if you have been advised to take a full course. Ring your doctor for advice if you need to stop for any reason. Some drugs have to be stopped gradually rather than abruptly.

8. Be on the look out for side-effects and remember that if you seem to develop new symptoms while taking a prescription drug then the chances are high that the new symptoms were caused by the treatment you are taking for your original symptoms.

9. Report any side-effects to your doctor – and ask him if he's going to report the side-effects to the authorities. The vast majority of doctors never bother to report side-effects – with the result that potentially hazardous drugs remain on the market for far longer than they should.

10. If you need to see a doctor while taking a drug make sure he knows what you are taking – particularly if he intends to prescribe new treatment for you. Many drugs do not mix well together and may, indeed, react together in a dangerous way.

11. Do not assume that a doctor you have seen in the past will remember what he prescribed for you on a previous occasion.

12. Learn the names and purposes of the drugs you take. If you are not sure when to take the drugs that you have been given ask your doctor or the pharmacist. If you think you will forget the instructions you are given ask for them to be written down. The name of the drug should always appear on the container.

13. Do not remove drugs from their proper containers except when you need them or if you are transferring them to a device intended to help you remember to take them.

14. Try to see the same doctor as often as possible. If several doctors are prescribing for you there is an increased risk of an interaction between drugs which do not mix well.

15. Use drugs with care and caution, but do use them when they are required. Doctors sometimes divide patients into two main groups: those who are willing to take drugs for any little symptom and who feel deprived if not offered a pharmacological solution to every ailment, and those who are unwilling to take drugs under any circumstances. Try not to fall into either of these extremist groups.

DON'T BE DISAPPOINTED IF YOUR DOCTOR DOESN'T PRESCRIBE FOR YOU

Doctors sometimes argue that they only overprescribe because of pressure from patients to do so. If, when you visit your doctor, he doesn't give you any pills, be pleased! And if he does give you a prescription, check that the drug is really necessary and that your doctor isn't giving the drug to you because he thinks you want it.

TWELVE COMMON SIDE-EFFECTS TO WATCH OUT FOR

1. Drowsiness is a common problem with all drugs which have an effect on the central nervous system – these include sedatives, tranquillisers, sleeping pills, most drugs used in the treatment of anxiety and depression, and drugs used in the treatment of epilepsy. Drowsiness is also common with antihistamines (these are commonly used for allergies and so patients suffering from hay fever should be aware that their medication may make them feel sleepy).

2. Nausea and vomiting are caused by many different drugs including pain relievers, drugs used to treat infections, hormones and drugs prescribed for heart conditions.

3. Dizziness is commonly caused by aspirin but drugs used to treat high blood pressure, nerve disorders such as anxiety and depression and infections can also cause this side effect.

4. Drugs such as penicillin which are used to treat infection, often cause diarrhoea – as do some drugs prescribed for intestinal disorders such as indigestion, gastritis and constipation.

5. Headache is a symptom that is associated with a huge range of drugs.

6. Drugs used in the treatment of high blood pressure and in the treatment of nerve problems are particularly likely to produce a dry mouth.

7. Pain relievers, drugs used to treat infections and steroid drugs are the prescription products which are most likely to cause indigestion or wind.

8. Skin rashes are extremely common among patients taking drugs. Drugs used to treat infections – such as penicillin and sulphonamide – are commonly associated with this problem. A skin rash may suggest an allergy to a drug.

9. Itching associated with a skin rash means that an allergy reaction is very likely.

10. Constipation is a common side effect with pain relievers, antacids, cough medicines and (naturally enough) drugs used in the treatment of diarrhoea.

11. Other side-effects which are commonly noticed by patients taking prescription drugs include: confusion, hallucinations, tremors, fainting, wheezing, palpitations, blurred vision, depression, sweating, ringing in the ears and sexual problems such as frigidity and impotence.

12. Remember: you can develop virtually any side effect with virtually any drug. If you do develop side-effects it is vitally important that you speak to your doctor before you stop taking your medication. Always follow your doctor's advice about how and when to take a drug – and if you are in any doubt then ask for a second opinion.

HOW TO TELL IF YOUR DOCTOR IS TRYING OUT A NEW DRUG ON YOU

Every week thousands of patients are used – often unwittingly – in medical experiments. Doctors in general practice and in hospitals – make a great deal of money testing new drugs for pharmaceutical companies. But patients are often put at risk unnecessarily. Be suspicious if your doctor makes a great fuss of you, is unusually polite or wants you to return to the clinic at very regular intervals.

If instead of handing you a prescription, your doctor gives you a bottle of pills and doesn't charge you for them then the pills may be new and you may be taking part in a drug trial.

Watch out if your doctor asks you a lot of questions that don't seem entirely relevant. If your doctor is doing a clinical trial for a drug company he will almost certainly ask you lots of questions about side-effects – questions that he would not normally ask.

Be wary if your doctor wants you to undergo blood or other tests but doesn't explain why the tests are necessary. Drug companies paying for new drugs to be tested may want blood tests performed.

If your doctor admits that he wants to try out a new drug on you make sure that there is no existing alternative. New drugs should only be tried out on patients when there are no effective and safe alternatives. Why should you risk your health (and your life) to benefit your doctor's bank balance and the drug company's profits?

SENSITIVITY REACTIONS

Some patients cannot take some drugs without coming out in a red, itchy rash and/or developing other signs of sensitivity. Penicillin is one of the drugs most commonly associated with this type of allergy reaction.

Once a patient has shown unequivocal signs of a drug allergy care should be taken not to expose the patient to that drug again. A second reaction may be more serious.

The patient's doctor will normally make a note on the medical records but it may also be wise to invest in a special bracelet or necklace upon which details of your problem can be engraved. (Your doctor or pharmacist should have details.)

DRUGS THAT WERE SO DANGEROUS THEY HAD TO BE BANNED

During the last three decades over 70 prescription drugs have been withdrawn from sale because it was feared that they were not safe for patients to use.

The top categories of drugs which are withdrawn because of fears about their safety include:

a) drugs used in the treatment of arthritis

b) pain-killers

c) antidepressants

Before 1983 an average of just 2.2 drugs per year were withdrawn from sale. But since 1983 the number of drugs withdrawn from sale has increased to an average of 8.6 a year!

Drugs are not always withdrawn from sale at the same time in different countries. One drug which was first used at the beginning of the century was officially withdrawn in different countries between 1970 and 1986!

THE TOP TEN PRESCRIPTION GROUPS

Drugs acting on the nervous system – including sleeping tablets, pain-killers and anxiety pills – are the most popularly prescribed drugs.

Here are the top ten groups of prescription drugs:

1. Drugs acting on the nervous system

2. Antibiotics such as penicillin

3. Respiratory tract drugs such as cough medicines

4. Heart drugs

5. Drugs acting on stomach and bowels

6. Skin preparations

7. Products such as iron and vitamin tablets

8. Ear, nose and throat preparations

9. Drugs used in the treatment of rheumatic diseases

10. Drugs acting on the metabolism – including hormones

(This list refers to therapeutic drugs – otherwise the contraceptive pill would figure prominently).

DRUGS DON'T ALWAYS MIX WELL

Many drugs do not mix well together and may indeed react together in a dangerous way. Since a large number of patients regularly take two or more drugs this is a real problem. Patients already taking prescribed drugs who are offered prescriptions for additional products should ask their doctor to confirm that the drugs will not interact badly. Patients taking prescribed drugs should not take drugs bought over the counter unless they have been assured by their doctor and/or pharmacist that the combination will be entirely safe.

RED IS FOR PAIN!

Drug companies have found that patients with different illnesses respond best to tablets which are a particular colour. Patients who are in pain seem to get the best relief from pills which are coloured red. Patients who are anxious or depressed often seem to respond best to drugs which are coloured yellow or green.

TIPS FOR PATIENTS TAKING ANTIBIOTICS

It is usually important to take antibiotics until the bottle is empty. If half a course is taken then there is a risk that the infection will come back. If side-effects develop contact your doctor. He will have to decide whether or not the course of antibiotics should be completed – despite the side-effects.

DRUGS AND CHILDREN

Children are not just miniature adults, and they do not always metabolise drugs in the same way that adults do. This means that the popular practice of simply reducing the adult dose of a drug when prescribing it for a child is not a particularly sensible one. Unfortunately, many of the drugs available today have not been effectively tested on children, and there is often no information available to enable practitioners to judge precisely how and what to prescribe.

It is, for this reason, particularly important to ensure that children are only given drugs when no alternative form of treatment is available.

Some children have difficulty in swallowing tablets or capsules and this problem can occasionally be overcome by hiding the tablets in small quantities of a favourite food offered on a teaspoon. Tablets should not be crushed and capsules should not be opened before being taken since such action may affect the safety and effectiveness of the product.

It is important to check with your doctor and/or pharmacist before giving drugs with food since the effectiveness of some medications may be adversely affected if they are taken with food.

DRUGS THAT ARE USELESS

Every day millions of prescriptions are written for medicines which will be of little or no practical value – and which, on balance, will probably do more harm than good. Examples include:

1. Cough medicines are rarely powerful enough to suppress coughing – and since coughing helps bring infected material out of the lungs that is probably just as well. However, patients swallow millions of gallons of the stuff every year.

2. Sleeping tablets are taken by millions and are a major source of revenue for the drug companies. But if taken for more than a few weeks many sleeping tablets can be addictive and may start to induce sleeplessness! (A phenomenon which explains why so many people on sleeping pills gradually increase their night-time dosage in a vain attempt to get to sleep.)

3. Antibiotics are of no value when prescribed for patients suffering from viral infections (unless there is a risk of another, bacterial infection developing) but many doctors routinely prescribe antibiotics for colds and flu – which are caused by viruses. It has been estimated that 50% of the prescriptions written for antibiotics are a waste of time and money.

STORING MEDICINES

Medicines should be stored in the containers in which they were supplied and the labels should not be removed. Containers should be kept tightly fastened and out of extremes of both heat and cold. If there is an expiry date on a prescription medicine then the medicine should either be returned to the pharmacy or safely disposed of on or after that date.

Any prescribed medicines not needed on a regular basis should be thrown away without delay. Any medicine that changes in appearance should be discarded.

Many drug packages now contain an expiry date but if there is no official expiry date it is usually safest to assume that drugs should be thrown away when they are six months old.

SIDE-EFFECTS WHICH ARE COMMONER AMONG ELDERLY PATIENTS

Patients who are over the age of 65 are more likely to suffer from side-effects when taking drugs. This is because as the human body gets older it becomes less efficient at dealing with drugs – and more sensitive. Drug companies and doctors often recommend that older patients should be given reduced dosages of pills.

1. Drowsiness and confusion are commoner among the elderly after taking sleeping tablets or tranquillisers.

2. Dizziness, lightheadedness and fainting and falling are commoner among the elderly when they take drugs to treat high blood pressure.

3. Constipation after taking a pain killer is commoner among the elderly.

4. Stomach upsets – including ulceration – are commoner after taking drugs for the management of arthritis.

5. Problems in passing urine may be commoner among the elderly when they need to take drugs.

TAKING DRUGS DURING BREAST-FEEDING

The increase in the number of women breast-feeding their babies is matched by the increase in the number of different drugs taken by new mothers. Although some drugs may well have no effect on the newborn baby and may not be excreted in the breast-milk, I believe that caution is sensible. The amount of evidence on this subject is very slight.

In general, I would recommend that no mother should breast-feed while taking a drug unless assured by her own GP or by the doctor looking after her that it is safe for her to do so.

ADVICE FOR PREGNANT WOMEN

Pregnant women are doubly vulnerable when taking prescription drugs – both they and their unborn child may be at risk. Some drugs are more likely than others to cause problems in the womb. Women who are pregnant – or who think they might or could be pregnant – should always tell their doctor if he is planning to prescribe for them. The most critical period for an unborn baby is the first three months of its life – a point at which its mother may not even know of its existence. It is during this period that the baby is developing most rapidly and is, therefore, most vulnerable to outside change.

No pregnant woman should take any drug or medicine unless it has been prescribed for her by a doctor who knows that she is pregnant. This means that a woman on long-term medication who becomes pregnant must revisit her doctor straight away, that no woman should take a drug prescribed by a doctor who may not be aware that she is pregnant and that no pregnant woman should take any home medicine without permission from her doctor.

An authoritative report has concluded that "it is impossible to prove beyond a shadow of a doubt that any drug is absolutely safe in pregnancy" and that "drugs should not be given during pregnancy unless they are essential".

Incidentally, some particularly cautious doctors assume that all women of child-bearing age are pregnant until proved otherwise and may refuse to prescribe until reassured on this point.

A TIP FOR PATIENTS TAKING PILLS

Always take pills with a full glass of water. This will help make sure that the tablet, capsule or pill goes down successfully. It is easier to take a pill if you are standing up rather than sitting down.

TIPS TO HELP AVOID GETTING HOOKED ON A TRANQUILLISER

The risk of benzodiazepine-related dependence may be minimised by adopting the following guidelines for treatment:

1. Patients should take benzodiazepines for short periods – or intermittently.

2. The lowest possible dose should be used.

3. The doctor should review treatment regularly; and especially before repeating prescriptions.

4. Treatment should be discontinued gradually, taking into account patient reaction at each stage.

The risk of dependence increases with higher doses and longer-term use and is further increased in patients with a history of alcoholism, drug abuse or in patients with marked personality disorders.

Symptoms such as anxiety, depression, headache, insomnia, tension and sweating have been reported following abrupt discontinuation of benzodiazepines and these symptoms may be difficult to distinguish from the original symptoms of anxiety. Other symptoms such as persistent tinnitus, involuntary movements, paraesthesia, perceptual changes, confusion, convulsions, abdominal and muscle cramps and vomiting may be characteristic of benzodiazepine withdrawal syndrome.

LIQUID MEDICINES

When liquids are prescribed it is important to shake the bottle before pouring out the recommended dose, since some liquid preparations may separate during storage.

Do not drink medicine straight from the bottle. Infections can easily be transmitted this way. Use a spoon or measuring cup so that you can be sure you take the correct dose.

TIPS FOR PATIENTS TRYING TO COME OFF TRANQUILLISERS

During the last few decades it has become clear that millions of patients have become addicted to tranquillisers and sleeping tablets. It isn't always easy to get off these drugs. Here are some tips that should help.

1. Visit your doctor and ask for his or her help. If you do not receive sympathetic support then change doctors.

2. It is important to reduce your dose slowly in order to minimise the withdrawal symptoms. The length of time it will take you to stop your pills will depend on the dose you were taking and how long you were taking the drugs.

3. Remember that when you do stop the pills your original symptoms – the symptoms for which you took the drugs – will probably return.

NOT ALL DRUGS ARE TAKEN BY MOUTH – OR EVEN BY INJECTION!

Traditionally, most drugs are taken by mouth or given by injection. In recent years, however, the popularity of other types of presentation has increased. For example, an increasing number of patients now take their drugs in suppository form. This has for many years been an accepted route in France. The main advantage is that stomach upsets are completely avoided.

Even more recently there has been a dramatic increase in the interest shown in products designed to be used through the skin. There are now products available as creams and ointments designed to have an effect on the whole body. Hormones, for example, seem particularly suitable for this type of preparation. It seems very likely that in the future a considerable amount of research will be done on drug presentation as well as drug content. Patients should be prepared to receive prescriptions for drugs designed to be used in rather unusual ways.

WHAT YOU SHOULD KNOW ABOUT REPEAT PRESCRIPTIONS

A growing number of prescriptions (now said to be about half of all those written) are provided without there being any meeting between the doctor and the patient. The patient writes or telephones for a new supply of a specific drug and then , a day or so later, either collects or receives through the post the appropriate prescription.

This system of providing prescriptions "on request" was originally designed to help patients suffering from chronic disorders such as diabetes, high blood pressure or epilepsy. Patients suffering from disorders which tend to vary very little over the months do not need regular medical examinations but they do need supplies of drugs. For them to have to visit a doctor simply to obtain a prescription is a waste of everyone's time. Doctors do not usually prescribe quantities of drugs likely to last more than four to six weeks since some drugs deteriorate if kept too long and most practitioners feel that it is unwise to allow any patient to keep excessively large quantities of drugs at home.

Unfortunately, repeat prescribing is not always restricted to patients with long-term problems requiring continuous medication. Patients who really should see a doctor rather than continue taking tablets sometimes ask for repeat prescriptions and, to the shame of the medical profession, not infrequently obtain them. Many patients have become psychologically dependent on sleeping tablets and tranquillisers because of the ease with which they have been able to obtain repeat prescriptions.

Arrangements for obtaining repeat prescriptions vary a good deal from practice to practice. In some practices patients entitled to receive prescriptions are issued with cards on which the drugs which they are allowed to receive without any consultation are listed. There may be a limit on the number of prescriptions which any patient may obtain without being reviewed. In other practices the cards detailing drugs which can be provided on repeat prescriptions are kept with the patient's notes so that the receptionists, who usually write out repeat prescriptions, can check on drugs and dosages, and make a note of the number of prescriptions used.

Theoretically, doctors signing prescriptions should check all the details, including specific points such as the dosages and quantities of drugs to be supplied, and general points such as the suitability of continuing with the treatment. In practice, many prescriptions supplied in this way are signed almost without the doctor looking at them.

For this reason I suggest that patients receiving drugs on repeat prescriptions should always check that the tablets they receive match the tablets previously prescribed and that any instructions on the bottle label match previous instructions. If there is any confusion or uncertainty then an urgent telephone call should be made to the surgery.

As a general rule, I suggest that only patients who have established and long-term clinical problems should obtain drugs on repeat prescriptions and they should visit the surgery at least once every six months to check that the medication does not need changing. Patients with short-term or acute conditions who need medication should always speak to a doctor.

QUESTIONS TO ASK YOUR DOCTOR BEFORE TAKING A DRUG

Patients have a right to know what they are taking – and why. Don't be shy. Here are some questions you should ask your doctor:

1. What is this medicine for?

2. How long should I take it? Should I take it until the bottle is empty or until my symptoms have gone?

3. What should I do if I miss a dose?

4. What side-effects should I particularly watch out for? Will it make me drowsy?

5. Am I likely to need to take more when these have gone? Should I arrange another consultation?

6. Are there any foods I should avoid? Should I take it before, with or after food? Should I avoid alcohol?

7. How long will the medicine take to work – and how will I know that it is working?

TIPS FOR WOMEN TAKING THE CONTRACEPTIVE PILL

1. You must have regular check ups if you are taking the contraceptive pill. You should visit your doctor at least once every six months – more often if he advises it.

2. If you have been taking the contraceptive pill for several years ask your doctor whether it is safe for you to continue.

3. See your doctor immediately if you notice symptoms such as: severe pain or swelling in the calf; chest pains; stomach pains; breathlessness; fainting; fits; speech defects; an inability to see clearly; any unexplained or unexpected bleeding; any sudden numbing or weakness; jaundice; any generalised skin rash; headache; or any other recurrent, persistent or worrying symptom.

4. Contraceptive pills do not always mix well with other drugs. Check with your doctor if you need to take any other drugs while taking the contraceptive pill.

5. If you want to get pregnant, I suggest that you stop your pill six months in advance to give your own hormones a chance to get back to normal.

6. Do not breast-feed while taking a contraceptive pill – the hormones could get through to your breast-milk.

7. If you suffer an intestinal upset – for example, a bout of diarrhoea – check with your doctor. You may not be protected and may need to take other precautions to avoid pregnancy.

NOT ALL DRUGS WORK!

Drug companies only have to provide evidence that their drugs are safe before they can obtain marketing licences; they do not have to produce any really objective evidence that they work.

Inevitably this means that a large number of inefficient, ineffective drugs are available on prescription. Many of these drugs rely on the 'placebo effect' for any value they may have.

WHAT'S IN A NAME?

Note: Many patients get confused when they are given a prescription for a drug and notice that the name is different. This may be a mistake (so check) but doctors do often prescribe drugs by two names – a general or generic name (given to all versions of the drug) and a brand name (given to one company's version of that drug).

Although the World Health Organisation has estimated that few prescribers need more than 200 drugs in their armamentarium, there are many thousands of drug products on the market. There are considerably more than 20,000 drugs available.

A great many of these products are virtually identical in chemical value. There are, for example, scores of indigestion remedies containing the same basic ingredients, dozens of antibiotics with similar properties, and a great many pain-killers, contraceptive pills, sleeping tablets and tranquillisers. Doctors choosing which product to prescribe have much the same sort of problem as customers in a pharmacy trying to decide which headache remedy to choose.

The number of genuinely different, 'new' drugs introduced onto the market each year is very small. The number of alternative drugs introduced is enormous.

Every drug that a doctor prescribes will fall into one of two groups: branded and generic. The term *generic* simply means that the name is a general one describing a kind of pharmacological product and is not associated with any particular manufacturer.

Because the drug companies usually manage to give their products names that are shorter and easier to remember than the generic names, most doctors prescribe branded products rather than generic products. The drug companies claim that this is wise because branded products are made according to strict regulations. Others argue that branded products are nearly always more expensive than generic products and that the regulations governing the manufacture of generic products are strict enough to ensure that there is little practical difference between a generic product and a branded product.

TESTED ON ANIMALS

Although there are no laws demanding that they do so, pharmaceutical companies tend to test all their drugs on animals. Many people who strongly object to the use of animals in experiments worry that this means they should not take prescription drugs, however ill they may be. However, since animal experiments are pointless and do NOT contribute to the development of new drugs in any way, I do not believe that anyone should refuse drug therapy for this reason.

There is an analysis of the use of animals in laboratory experiments and evidence supporting my claim that such experiments are pointless, in my book *Betrayal of Trust* published by the European Medical Journal. One of my other books *Why Animal Experiments Must Stop* (same publisher), also deals with this subject in considerable detail.

ARE YOU TAKING A PLACEBO?

Approximately one-third of all patients will obtain relief from tablets and medicines which contain absolutely no pharmacologically active constituents and which work by intent rather than by any immediately discernible physiological effect.

Even patients suffering from severe pain have benefited from the so-called placebo effect, and dozens of reliable studies have shown that patients suffering genuine discomfort have obtained noticeable relief from the use of sugar tablets.

Recent research has shown that when a placebo is taken a special hormone seems to be released by the brain. This hormone is part of the body's own internal defence mechanism and it seems likely that the placebo pill is simply triggering an automatic release of a pain-relieving product. Since placebos only work when the patient believes that they will work, the placebo effect is more marked among anxious, rather dependent individuals than among strong-willed, self-sufficient, suspicious people.

Those who oppose the use of placebos claim that to deceive the patient is wrong even if he benefits, and that there is a real risk of turning a healthy patient into a hypochondriac by giving him a placebo.

Those who favour the use of placebos claim that even some of our most pharmacologically effective drugs frequently do their job because of the placebo reaction, and that, whether doctors and patients recognise it or not, between one-third and one half of all prescriptions are given partly or wholly for their placebo effect. The use of an inert, inactive product as a placebo is defended on the grounds that a substance which contains no active ingredients will be unlikely to produce any side-effects. (It is worth remembering that four out of ten patients who take prescription drugs will suffer noticeable or potentially lethal side-effects.)

DRUGS NEED TO BE TAKEN WITH PRECISION

It is a sad but true fact that of all the drugs prescribed only a relatively small number are taken in the way that the prescriber originally intended them to be taken. Drugs are taken at the wrong time, they are taken with food when they should be taken before or after food, they are forgotten, they are taken too frequently and they are sometimes never taken out of the bottle at all.

It is important to remember that modern prescribed drugs are not only potentially effective but also powerful and potentially dangerous. Drug companies spend a considerable amount of money on refining their manufacturing process and on ensuring that the drugs they make will be made available to the appropriate tissues within the body at a suitable rate. Taking pills at the wrong time or in the wrong way can render such careful preparation useless.

There are several questions which should be answered before a patient starts taking a drug. Usually the answers to these questions will appear on the label of the bottle containing the drugs. If the answers do not appear there then the fault may lie with the doctor who wrote the prescription or the pharmacist who dispensed it.

Here are some things to watch out for:

1. Some drugs can be stopped when symptoms cease. Others need to be taken as a complete course. A small number of drugs need to be taken continuously and a second prescription will have to be obtained before the first supply has run out. The patient who knows what his drug is for, why he is taking it and what the effect should be, will be more likely to know when a drug is to be stopped.

2. If a drug has to be taken once a day, it does not usually matter what time of day it is taken, as long as it is taken at the same time each day. If a drug has to be taken twice a day it should be taken at intervals of 12 hours. A drug that needs to be taken three times a day should be taken at eight-hourly intervals and a drug that needs taking four times a day should be taken at six-hourly intervals. The day should be divided into suitable segments.

3. Some drugs which may cause stomach problems are safer when taken with meals. Other drugs may not be absorbed properly if taken with food. Always check with your doctor and/or pharmacist. It is also important to remember that many drugs may interact dangerously if alcohol is drunk.

4. A number of patients (particularly the elderly) are expected to remember to take dozens of pills a day. When a day's medication includes tablets to be taken twice daily, three times daily, mornings only and every four hours, mistakes are inevitable. If a patient needs to take a number of drugs a day, mistakes can be minimised by preparing a daily chart on which the names and times of different drugs are marked. Such a chart will reduce the risk of a patient taking one dose twice or struggling to remember whether a particular pill has yet been taken.

5. To avoid the risk of overdosage, sleeping tablets should not be kept by the bedside. It is too easy for a half-asleep patient to take extra tablets in error. In the case of a suspected overdose, medical attention must be sought.

PART TWO

THE DRUGS

AN A-Z LIST OF COMMONLY PRESCRIBED DRUGS

ACEPRIL

POSSIBLE REASONS TO TAKE IT MAY INCLUDE: For the treatment of mild to moderate hypertension and congestive heart failure and following myocardial infarction.

HOW IS IT PRESCRIBED: Usually twice or three times a day.

POSSIBLE SIDE-EFFECTS MAY INCLUDE: Angioedema involving the extremities, face lips, mucous membranes, tongue, glottis or larynx; neutropenia, anaemia and thrombocytopenia; proteinuria, elevated blood urea and creatinine, elevated serum potassium and acidosis, hypotension and tachycardia. Skin rashes, usually pruritic, may occur – these are usually mild, maculopapular, rarely urticarial and disappear within a few days of dosage reduction, short-term treatment with an antihistamine and/or discontinuing therapy. In a few cases the rash has been associated with fever. Pruritus, flushing, vesicular or bullous rash, photosensitivity; self-limiting taste impairment, weight loss may be associated with the loss of taste; stomatitis, resembling aphthous ulcers; elevation of liver enzymes; gastric irritation, abdominal pain.

WARNING
You should call your doctor immediately if you develop any side effect while taking a drug. If you do develop side-effects it is vitally important that you speak to your doctor before you stop taking your pills. Remember that this list of side-effects isn't complete – you can develop virtually any side effect with virtually any drug – and remember too that some of these side-effects are quite uncommon and many patients can take a drug without getting any side-effects. Always follow your doctor's advice about how and when to take a drug – and if you are in any doubt at all then ask for a second opinion. The fact that one drug may be accompanied by a long list of possible side-effects does not mean that it is necessarily more or less dangerous or more or less likely to produce problems than a drug which has a shorter list of possible side-effects.

ACHROMYCIN

POSSIBLE REASONS TO TAKE IT MAY INCLUDE: For the treatment of infections – including chest infections and acne.

HOW IS IT PRESCRIBED: Usually four times a day.

POSSIBLE SIDE-EFFECTS MAY INCLUDE: Nausea, vomiting, diarrhoea, skin problems, raised intracranial pressure.

ACICLOVIR TABLETS

POSSIBLE REASONS TO TAKE IT MAY INCLUDE: For the treatment of herpes simplex virus infections of the skin and mucous membranes including initial and recurrent genital herpes.

HOW IS IT PRESCRIBED: Tablets should usually be taken five times daily at approximately four-hourly intervals omitting the night-time dose. Treatment should continue for five days, but in severe initial infections this may have to be extended.

POSSIBLE SIDE-EFFECTS MAY INCLUDE: Skin rashes; gastro-intestinal effects including nausea, vomiting, diarrhoea and abdominal pains; reversible neurological reactions, notably dizziness, confusional states, hallucinations and somnolence; accelerated diffuse hair loss; mild, transient rises in bilirubin and liver-related enzymes, small increases in blood urea and creatinine, small decreases in haemotological indices; headaches.

ADALAT RETARD

POSSIBLE REASONS TO TAKE IT MAY INCLUDE: For the treatment of hypertension and the prophylaxis of angina pectoris.

HOW IS IT PRESCRIBED: Usually one tablet twice-daily.

POSSIBLE SIDE-EFFECTS MAY INCLUDE: Headache, flushing, tachycardia, palpitations, gravitational oedema; paraesthesia, dizziness, lethargy, rash, pruritus, urticaria.

ADIFAX

POSSIBLE REASONS TO TAKE IT MAY INCLUDE: To help weight loss in severe obesity.

HOW IS IT PRESCRIBED: Usually twice a day.

POSSIBLE SIDE-EFFECTS MAY INCLUDE: Dry mouth, nausea, constipation, diarrhoea, drowsiness, dizziness, urinary frequency, headache, mood disturbances, weakness, insomnia, symptoms of depression, nervousness and conjunctivitis.

ADIZEM

POSSIBLE REASONS TO TAKE IT MAY INCLUDE: Management of angina pectoris and treatment of mild to moderate hypertension.

HOW IS IT PRESCRIBED: Usually three times a day.

POSSIBLE SIDE-EFFECTS MAY INCLUDE: Nausea, headache, skin rashes, oedema of the legs, flushing, hypotension, fatigue, bradycardia, changes in liver function tests and renal function.

AEROLIN AUTOHALER

POSSIBLE REASONS TO TAKE IT MAY INCLUDE: For the treatment of asthma and similar conditions.

HOW IS IT PRESCRIBED: Available as a breath-actuated metered-dose aerosol.

POSSIBLE SIDE-EFFECTS MAY INCLUDE: Fine muscle tremor, headache, increase in heart rate, muscle cramps.

ALLOPURINOL

POSSIBLE REASONS TO TAKE IT MAY INCLUDE: For the treatment of gout and renal stones.

HOW IS IT PRESCRIBED: The dosage is adjusted by monitoring serum urate concentrations and urinary urate/uric acid levels.

POSSIBLE SIDE-EFFECTS MAY INCLUDE: Skin reactions may be pruritic, maculopapular, sometimes scaly, sometimes purpuric and rarely exfoliative; fever, lymphadenopathy, arthralgia and/or eosinophilia resembling Stevens-Johnson and/or Lyell Syndrome; hepatitis, interstitial nephritis, epilepsy; angioimmunoblastic lymphadenopathy; granulomatous hepatitis, without overt evidence of more generalised hypersensitivity; nausea and vomiting; recurrent haematemesis, steatorrhoea; thrombocytopenia, agranulocytosis and aplastic anaemia; fever, general malaise, asthenia, headache, vertigo, ataxia, somnolence, coma, depression, paralysis, paraesthesiae, neuropathy, visual disorder, cataract, macular changes, taste perversion, stomatitis, changed bowel habit, infertility, impotence, nocturnal emision, diabetes mellitus, hyperlipaemia, furunculosis, alopecia, discoloured hair, angina, hypertension, bradycardia, oedema, uraemia, haematuria, gynaecomastia.

WARNING

You should call your doctor immediately if you develop any side effect while taking a drug. If you do develop side-effects it is vitally important that you speak to your doctor before you stop taking your pills. Remember that this list of side-effects isn't complete – you can develop virtually any side effect with virtually any drug – and remember too that some of these side-effects are quite uncommon and many patients can take a drug without getting any side-effects. Always follow your doctor's advice about how and when to take a drug – and if you are in any doubt at all then ask for a second opinion. The fact that one drug may be accompanied by a long list of possible side-effects does not mean that it is necessarily more or less dangerous or more or less likely to produce problems than a drug which has a shorter list of possible side-effects.

ALU-CAP

POSSIBLE REASONS TO TAKE IT MAY INCLUDE: For the treatment of too much stomach acid.

HOW IS IT PRESCRIBED: Usually around four times a day.

POSSIBLE SIDE-EFFECTS MAY INCLUDE: Constipation.

ALUDROX

POSSIBLE REASONS TO TAKE IT MAY INCLUDE: For the treatment of peptic ulceration, dyspepsia, too much stomach acid.

HOW IS IT PRESCRIBED: Usually around four times a day.

POSSIBLE SIDE-EFFECTS MAY INCLUDE: Constipation.

ALUMINIUM HYDROXIDE

POSSIBLE REASONS TO TAKE IT MAY INCLUDE: For the treatment of peptic ulceration, dyspepsia, too much stomach acid.

HOW IS IT PRESCRIBED: Usually around four times a day.

POSSIBLE SIDE-EFFECTS MAY INCLUDE: Constipation.

AMFIPEN

POSSIBLE REASONS TO TAKE IT MAY INCLUDE: For the treatment of a wide range of infections caused by ampicillin-sensitive organisms.

HOW IS IT PRESCRIBED: Usually four times daily.

POSSIBLE SIDE-EFFECTS MAY INCLUDE: Pseudomembranous colitis; skin reactions may be due to either penicillin hypersensitivity (urticarial rash) or specific ampicillin sensitivity (erythematous rash); diarrhoea. Superinfection by resistant organisms may occur following prolonged use.

AMITRIPTYLINE

POSSIBLE REASONS TO TAKE IT MAY INCLUDE: For the treatment of depression in adults.

HOW IS IT PRESCRIBED: Usually one tablet or capsule last thing at night. It is also available as injection and syrup.

POSSIBLE SIDE-EFFECTS MAY INCLUDE: Dry mouth, blurred vision, dizziness, fainting, drowsiness, nausea, vomiting, appetite loss, diarrhoea, constipation, difficulty in passing urine, tiredness, headache, hair loss, palpitations, sweating, tremors, rashes, confusion, disorientation, nightmares, delusions, restlessness, hallucinations, convulsions, sexual problems and irregular heart rhythms. Sudden withdrawal has been reported to cause nausea, headache and malaise.

AMLODIPINE

POSSIBLE REASONS TO TAKE IT MAY INCLUDE: For the treatment of high blood pressure and heart pain.

HOW IS IT PRESCRIBED: Usually once a day

POSSIBLE SIDE-EFFECTS MAY INCLUDE: Oedema, headache, nausea, fatigue, flushing, dizziness.

WARNING

You should call your doctor immediately if you develop any side effect while taking a drug. If you do develop side-effects it is vitally important that you speak to your doctor before you stop taking your pills. Remember that this list of side-effects isn't complete – you can develop virtually any side effect with virtually any drug – and remember too that some of these side-effects are quite uncommon and many patients can take a drug without getting any side-effects. Always follow your doctor's advice about how and when to take a drug – and if you are in any doubt at all then ask for a second opinion. The fact that one drug may be accompanied by a long list of possible side-effects does not mean that it is necessarily more or less dangerous or more or less likely to produce problems than a drug which has a shorter list of possible side-effects.

AMOXIL

POSSIBLE REASONS TO TAKE IT MAY INCLUDE: For the treatment of many different infections – including those affecting the chest, the bladder and the ear.

HOW IS IT PRESCRIBED: Commonly in capsule or tablet form, two or three times a day – but also available as a liquid or injection.

POSSIBLE SIDE-EFFECTS MAY INCLUDE: Diarrhoea, indigestion, skin rash.

AMOXYCILLIN

POSSIBLE REASONS TO TAKE IT MAY INCLUDE: For the treatment of many different infections – including those affecting the chest, the bladder and the ear.

HOW IS IT PRESCRIBED: Commonly in capsule or tablet form two or three times a day – but also available as a liquid or injection.

POSSIBLE SIDE-EFFECTS MAY INCLUDE: Diarrhoea, indigestion, skin rash.

APRINOX

POSSIBLE REASONS TO TAKE IT MAY INCLUDE: To get rid of fluid (prescribed for disorders as varied as swollen legs, heart failure and high blood pressure).

HOW IS IT PRESCRIBED: Usually mornings (so that you don't have to pass urine at night).

POSSIBLE SIDE-EFFECTS MAY INCLUDE: Dizziness, skin rashes, impotence, appetite loss, blood dyscrasias including agranulocytosis, aplastic anaemia, thrombocytopenia, leucopenia; pancreatitis.

ATENOLOL

POSSIBLE REASONS TO TAKE IT MAY INCLUDE: Management of hypertension, angina pectoris, cardiac arrhythmias, myocardial infarction.

HOW IS IT PRESCRIBED: Usually once or twice daily

POSSIBLE SIDE-EFFECTS MAY INCLUDE: Bradycardia, heart failure deterioration, postural hypotension which may be associated with syncope, cold extremities; precipitation of heart block, intermittent claudication, Raynaud's phenomenon; confusion, dizziness, headache, mood changes, nightmares, psychoses and hallucinations, sleep disturbances of the type noted with other beta-adrenoceptor blocking drugs; dry mouth, gastro-intestinal disturbances; purpura, thrombocytopenia; alopecia, dry eyes, psoriasiform skin reactions, exacerbation of psoriasis, skin rashes; paraesthesia; bronchospasm may occur in patients with bronchial asthma or a history of asthmatic complaints; visual disturbances; fatigue.

ATIVAN

POSSIBLE REASONS TO TAKE IT MAY INCLUDE: For the treatment of anxiety; recommended for short-term use of up to 4 weeks.

HOW IS IT PRESCRIBED: For moderate and severe anxiety commonly 1-4 mg daily in divided doses. As with all benzodiazepines long-term use may lead to dependence and withdrawal symptoms in certain patients. All patients taking Ativan should be carefully monitored and routine repeat prescriptions should be avoided. Treatment in all patients should be withdrawn gradually with careful monitoring and reassessment to minimise possible withdrawal symptoms. Patients who have taken benzodiazepines for a long time may require a longer period during which doses are reduced. The elderly may respond to lower doses and half the normal adult dose or less may be sufficient.

POSSIBLE SIDE-EFFECTS MAY INCLUDE: Daytime drowsiness; confusion, headache, dizziness, nausea, depression, change in appetite and sleep disturbance; blood dyscrasias and abnormal liver function tests; visual disturbances, hypotension, gastro-intestinal disturbances, skin rashes. The use of benzodiazepines may release suicidal tendencies in depressed patients. Ativan should not be used alone to treat depression.

WARNING

You should call your doctor immediately if you develop any side effect while taking a drug. If you do develop side-effects it is vitally important that you speak to your doctor before you stop taking your pills. Remember that this list of side-effects isn't complete – you can develop virtually any side effect with virtually any drug – and remember too that some of these side-effects are quite uncommon and many patients can take a drug without getting any side-effects. Always follow your doctor's advice about how and when to take a drug – and if you are in any doubt at all then ask for a second opinion. The fact that one drug may be accompanied by a long list of possible side-effects does not mean that it is necessarily more or less dangerous or more or less likely to produce problems than a drug which has a shorter list of possible side-effects.

AUGMENTIN

POSSIBLE REASONS TO TAKE IT MAY INCLUDE: For the treatment of infection.

HOW IS IT PRESCRIBED: Usually three times a day.

POSSIBLE SIDE-EFFECTS MAY INCLUDE: Diarrhoea, indigestion, nausea, vomiting, candidiasis, skin rash.

BECLOFORTE INHALER

POSSIBLE REASONS TO TAKE IT MAY INCLUDE: Prophylactic management of severe asthma.

HOW IS IT PRESCRIBED: Usually two inhalations (500 mg) twice daily, or one inhalation (250 mg) four times daily.

POSSIBLE SIDE-EFFECTS MAY INCLUDE: Candidiasis of the mouth and throat (thrush), the incidence increases with doses greater than 400 mg per day. Hoarseness or throat irritation; paradoxical bronchospasm may occur with an immediate increase in wheezing after dosing.

BECONASE AQUEOUS NASAL SPRAY

POSSIBLE REASONS TO TAKE IT MAY INCLUDE: The prophylaxis and treatment of perennial and seasonal allergic rhinitis, including hay fever.

HOW IS IT PRESCRIBED: Usually two sprays into each nostril twice daily.

POSSIBLE SIDE-EFFECTS MAY INCLUDE: Nasal septal perforation; dryness and irritation of the nose and throat, unpleasant taste and smell and epistaxis; raised intra-ocular pressure or glaucoma.

BECOTIDE INHALER

POSSIBLE REASONS TO TAKE IT MAY INCLUDE: For the management of asthma.

HOW IS IT PRESCRIBED: Dosage tailored for each patient.

POSSIBLE SIDE-EFFECTS MAY INCLUDE: Candidiasis of the mouth and throat (thrush); hoarseness or throat irritation; paradoxical bronchospasm may occur with an immediate increase in wheezing after dosing.

BENDROFLUAZIDE

POSSIBLE REASONS TO TAKE IT MAY INCLUDE: To get rid of fluid (prescribed for disorders as varied as swollen legs, heart failure and high blood pressure).

HOW IS IT PRESCRIBED: Usually mornings (so that you don't have to pass urine at night).

POSSIBLE SIDE-EFFECTS MAY INCLUDE: Dizziness, skin rashes, impotence, appetite loss, blood dyscrasias including agranulocytosis, aplastic anaemia, thrombocytopenia, leucopenia; pancreatitis.

BETA-PROGANE

POSSIBLE REASONS TO TAKE IT MAY INCLUDE: For the treatment of a wide range of conditions including heart pain, high blood pressure and anxiety.

HOW IS IT PRESCRIBED: Commonly one capsule morning or evening.

POSSIBLE SIDE-EFFECTS MAY INCLUDE: Cold extremities, nausea, diarrhoea, disturbed sleep, tiredness, hallucinations, skin rash, dry eyes.

WARNING

You should call your doctor immediately if you develop any side effect while taking a drug. If you do develop side-effects it is vitally important that you speak to your doctor before you stop taking your pills. Remember that this list of side-effects isn't complete – you can develop virtually any side effect with virtually any drug – and remember too that some of these side-effects are quite uncommon and many patients can take a drug without getting any side-effects. Always follow your doctor's advice about how and when to take a drug – and if you are in any doubt at all then ask for a second opinion. The fact that one drug may be accompanied by a long list of possible side-effects does not mean that it is necessarily more or less dangerous or more or less likely to produce problems than a drug which has a shorter list of possible side-effects.

BETIM

POSSIBLE REASONS TO TAKE IT MAY INCLUDE: For the treatment of high blood pressure, heart disease and migraine.

HOW IS IT PRESCRIBED: Usually once or twice a day.

POSSIBLE SIDE-EFFECTS MAY INCLUDE: Fatigue, weakness, heart failure, coldness of limb extremities, low blood pressure, heart block, epigastric distress, nausea, vomiting, dizziness, disorientation, vertigo, paraesthesia, headache, hallucinations, nightmares, insomnia, depression, breathing difficulty, skin rashes, dry eyes.

WARNING

You should call your doctor immediately if you develop any side effect while taking a drug. If you do develop side-effects it is vitally important that you speak to your doctor before you stop taking your pills. Remember that this list of side-effects isn't complete – you can develop virtually any side effect with virtually any drug – and remember too that some of these side-effects are quite uncommon and many patients can take a drug without getting any side-effects. Always follow your doctor's advice about how and when to take a drug – and if you are in any doubt at all then ask for a second opinion. The fact that one drug may be accompanied by a long list of possible side-effects does not mean that it is necessarily more or less dangerous or more or less likely to produce problems than a drug which has a shorter list of possible side-effects.

BETNOVATE

POSSIBLE REASONS TO TAKE IT MAY INCLUDE: For the treatment of eczema in children and adults but also in the treatment of a number of other skin conditions.

HOW IS IT PRESCRIBED: Usually a small quantity of Betnovate is applied to the affected area of skin two or three times daily until improvement occurs. It may then be possible to maintain improvement by applying once a day, or even less often, or by using a ready-diluted preparation.

POSSIBLE SIDE-EFFECTS MAY INCLUDE: Local atrophic changes in the skin such as striae, thinning, and dilation of the superficial blood vessels, particularly when occlusive dressings are used or when skin folds are involved. Prolonged use of large amounts or treatment of extensive areas can result in sufficient systemic absorption to produce the features of hypercorticism and suppression of the HPA axis. There are reports of pigmentation changes and hypertrichosis with topical steroids. Treatment of psoriasis with corticosteroids (or its withdrawal) is thought to have provoked the pustular form of the disease. Exacerbation of symptoms may occur.

WARNING
You should call your doctor immediately if you develop any side effect while taking a drug. If you do develop side-effects it is vitally important that you speak to your doctor before you stop taking your pills. Remember that this list of side-effects isn't complete – you can develop virtually any side effect with virtually any drug – and remember too that some of these side-effects are quite uncommon and many patients can take a drug without getting any side-effects. Always follow your doctor's advice about how and when to take a drug – and if you are in any doubt at all then ask for a second opinion. The fact that one drug may be accompanied by a long list of possible side-effects does not mean that it is necessarily more or less dangerous or more or less likely to produce problems than a drug which has a shorter list of possible side-effects.

BLOCADREN

POSSIBLE REASONS TO TAKE IT MAY INCLUDE: For the treatment of high blood pressure, heart disease and migraine.

HOW IS IT PRESCRIBED: Often once or twice a day.

POSSIBLE SIDE-EFFECTS MAY INCLUDE: Fatigue, weakness, heart failure, coldness of limb extremities, low blood pressure, heart block, nausea, vomiting, dizziness, vertigo, paraesthesia, hallucinations, nightmares, insomnia, depression, breathing difficulty, skin rashes, dry eyes.

BRICANYL INHALER

POSSIBLE REASONS TO TAKE IT MAY INCLUDE: For the treatment of bronchospasm in bronchial asthma and in chronic bronchitis, emphysema and other bronchopulmonary disorders in which bronchospasm is a complicating factor.

HOW IS IT PRESCRIBED: Prophylaxis and relief of acute attacks: one or two inhalations as required, with a short interval between each inhalation at six-hourly intervals.

POSSIBLE SIDE-EFFECTS MAY INCLUDE: Tremor, tonic cramp and palpitations; patients may feel tense; bronchospasm.

BRICANYL SA

POSSIBLE REASONS TO TAKE IT MAY INCLUDE: For the treatment of bronchospasm in bronchial asthma and in chronic bronchitis, emphysema and other bronchopulmonary disorders in which bronchospasm is a complicating factor.

HOW IS IT PRESCRIBED: Usually one tablet morning and evening. The tablet may not be divided or chewed, but must be swallowed whole together with liquid.

POSSIBLE SIDE-EFFECTS MAY INCLUDE: Tremor, headache, tonic cramp and palpitations; patients may feel tense; urticaria and exanthema may occur. In children, sleep disturbances and disturbances of behavioural effects have been observed.

WARNING
You should call your doctor immediately if you develop any side effect while taking a drug. If you do develop side-effects it is vitally important that you speak to your doctor before you stop taking your pills. Remember that this list of side-effects isn't complete – you can develop virtually any side effect with virtually any drug – and remember too that some of these side-effects are quite uncommon and many patients can take a drug without getting any side-effects. Always follow your doctor's advice about how and when to take a drug – and if you are in any doubt at all then ask for a second opinion. The fact that one drug may be accompanied by a long list of possible side-effects does not mean that it is necessarily more or less dangerous or more or less likely to produce problems than a drug which has a shorter list of possible side-effects.

BRITIAZIM

POSSIBLE REASONS TO TAKE IT MAY INCLUDE: For the management of angina pectoris.

HOW IS IT PRESCRIBED: Usually three times a day.

POSSIBLE SIDE-EFFECTS MAY INCLUDE: Nausea, headache, skin rashes, oedema of the ankles, flushing, bradycardia.

BRUFEN

POSSIBLE REASONS TO TAKE IT MAY INCLUDE: For the treatment of arthritis, rheumatoid arthritis, including juvenile rheumatoid arthritis, and soft-tissue injuries such as sprains and strains. Also prescribed for the relief of mild to moderate pain such as dysmenorrhoea, dental and post-operative pain and for the symptomatic relief of headache including migraine headache.

HOW IS IT PRESCRIBED: Recommended dosage for adults is 1200-1800 mg daily in divided doses. Some patients can be maintained on 600-1200 mg daily.

POSSIBLE SIDE-EFFECTS MAY INCLUDE: Nausea, vomiting, diarrhoea, dyspepsia, abdominal pain; skin rashes; thrombocytopenia.

WARNING
You should call your doctor immediately if you develop any side effect while taking a drug. If you do develop side-effects it is vitally important that you speak to your doctor before you stop taking your pills. Remember that this list of side-effects isn't complete – you can develop virtually any side effect with virtually any drug – and remember too that some of these side-effects are quite uncommon and many patients can take a drug without getting any side-effects. Always follow your doctor's advice about how and when to take a drug – and if you are in any doubt at all then ask for a second opinion. The fact that one drug may be accompanied by a long list of possible side-effects does not mean that it is necessarily more or less dangerous or more or less likely to produce problems than a drug which has a shorter list of possible side-effects.

BUCCASTEM

POSSIBLE REASONS TO TAKE IT MAY INCLUDE: For the treatment of vertigo, nausea, vomiting, migraine.

HOW IS IT PRESCRIBED: Usually twice a day.

POSSIBLE SIDE-EFFECTS MAY INCLUDE: Drowsiness, dizziness, skin reactions, dry mouth, agitation, insomnia.

BUMETANIDE

POSSIBLE REASONS TO TAKE IT MAY INCLUDE: Whenever diuretic therapy is required in the treatment of oedema, e.g. that associated with congestive heart failure, cirrhosis of the liver and renal disease including the nephrotic syndrome.

HOW IS IT PRESCRIBED: The 1 mg tablets are usually given as a single morning or early evening dose. Depending on the patient's response, a second dose can be given six to eight hours later.

POSSIBLE SIDE-EFFECTS MAY INCLUDE: Abdominal pain, vomiting, dyspepsia, diarrhoea, stomach and muscle cramps, arthralgia, dizziness, fatigue, hypotension, headache, nausea, encephalopathy (in patients with pre-existing hepatic disease), fluid and electrolyte depletion, dehydration, hyperuricemia, raised blood urea and serum creatinine, hyperglycaemia, abnormalities of serum levels of hepatic enzymes, skin rashes, pruritus, urticaria, thrombocytopenia, gynaecomastia and painful breasts.

WARNING

You should call your doctor immediately if you develop any side effect while taking a drug. If you do develop side-effects it is vitally important that you speak to your doctor before you stop taking your pills. Remember that this list of side-effects isn't complete – you can develop virtually any side effect with virtually any drug – and remember too that some of these side-effects are quite uncommon and many patients can take a drug without getting any side-effects. Always follow your doctor's advice about how and when to take a drug – and if you are in any doubt at all then ask for a second opinion. The fact that one drug may be accompanied by a long list of possible side-effects does not mean that it is necessarily more or less dangerous or more or less likely to produce problems than a drug which has a shorter list of possible side-effects.

BURINEX

POSSIBLE REASONS TO TAKE IT MAY INCLUDE: Whenever diuretic therapy is required in the treatment of oedema, e.g. that associated with congestive heart failure, cirrhosis of the liver and renal disease including the nephrotic syndrome.

HOW IS IT PRESCRIBED: The 1 mg tablets are usually given as a single morning or early evening dose. Depending on the patient's response, a second dose can be given six to eight hours later.

POSSIBLE SIDE-EFFECTS MAY INCLUDE: Abdominal pain, vomiting, dyspepsia, diarrhoea, stomach and muscle cramps, arthralgia, dizziness, fatigue, hypotension, headache, nausea, encephalopathy (in patients with pre-existing hepatic disease), fluid and electrolyte depletion, dehydration, hyperuricemia, raised blood urea and serum creatinine, hyperglycaemia, abnormalities of serum levels of hepatic enzymes, skin rashes, pruritus, urticaria, thrombocytopenia, gynaecomastia and painful breasts.

BUSPAR

POSSIBLE REASONS TO TAKE IT MAY INCLUDE: For the treatment of anxiety.

HOW IS IT PRESCRIBED: Two or three times a day.

POSSIBLE SIDE-EFFECTS MAY INCLUDE: Dizziness, headache, nervousness, tachycardia, chest pain, dry mouth, confusion, fatigue, light-headedness, excitement, nausea, sweating, drowsiness, palpitations.

BUSPIRONE

POSSIBLE REASONS TO TAKE IT MAY INCLUDE: For the treatment of anxiety.

HOW IS IT PRESCRIBED: Two or three times a day.

POSSIBLE SIDE-EFFECTS MAY INCLUDE: Dizziness, headache, nervousness, tachycardia, chest pain, dry mouth, confusion, fatigue, light-headedness, excitement, nausea, sweating, drowsiness, palpitations.

WARNING

You should call your doctor immediately if you develop any side effect while taking a drug. If you do develop side-effects it is vitally important that you speak to your doctor before you stop taking your pills. Remember that this list of side-effects isn't complete – you can develop virtually any side effect with virtually any drug – and remember too that some of these side-effects are quite uncommon and many patients can take a drug without getting any side-effects. Always follow your doctor's advice about how and when to take a drug – and if you are in any doubt at all then ask for a second opinion. The fact that one drug may be accompanied by a long list of possible side-effects does not mean that it is necessarily more or less dangerous or more or less likely to produce problems than a drug which has a shorter list of possible side-effects.

CALPOL

POSSIBLE REASONS TO TAKE IT MAY INCLUDE: For the treatment of mild to moderate pain (including teething pain) and as antipyretic in children.

HOW IS IT PRESCRIBED: Dosage tailored to the patient's age and needs.

POSSIBLE SIDE-EFFECTS MAY INCLUDE: Skin rashes and other allergic reactions; thrombocytopenic purpura, haemolytic anaemia and agranulocytosis; liver damage.

WARNING
You should call your doctor immediately if you develop any side effect while taking a drug. If you do develop side-effects it is vitally important that you speak to your doctor before you stop taking your pills. Remember that this list of side-effects isn't complete – you can develop virtually any side effect with virtually any drug – and remember too that some of these side-effects are quite uncommon and many patients can take a drug without getting any side-effects. Always follow your doctor's advice about how and when to take a drug – and if you are in any doubt at all then ask for a second opinion. The fact that one drug may be accompanied by a long list of possible side-effects does not mean that it is necessarily more or less dangerous or more or less likely to produce problems than a drug which has a shorter list of possible side-effects.

CANESTEN HC

POSSIBLE REASONS TO TAKE IT MAY INCLUDE: For the treatment of fungal infections.

HOW IS IT PRESCRIBED: Thinly and evenly applied to the affected area twice daily and rubbed in gently.

POSSIBLE SIDE-EFFECTS MAY INCLUDE: Local mild burning or irritation immediately after applying the cream. Hypersensitivity reactions may occur.

CAPOTEN

POSSIBLE REASONS TO TAKE IT MAY INCLUDE: For the treatment of mild to moderate hypertension and congestive heart failure and following myocardial infarction.

HOW IS IT PRESCRIBED: Usually twice or three times a day.

POSSIBLE SIDE-EFFECTS MAY INCLUDE: Angioedema involving the extremities, face lips, mucous membranes, tongue, glottis or larynx; neutropenia, anaemia and thrombocytopenia; proteinuria, elevated blood urea and creatinine, elevated serum potassium and acidosis, hypotension and tachycardia. Skin rashes, usually pruritic, may occur – these are usually mild, maculopapular, rarely urticarial and disappear within a few days of dosage reduction, short-term treatment with an antihistamine and/or discontinuing therapy. In a few cases the rash has been associated with fever. Pruritus, flushing, vesicular or bullous rash, photosensitivity; self-limiting taste impairment, weight loss may be associated with the loss of taste; stomatitis, resembling aphthous ulcers; elevation of liver enzymes; gastric irritation, abdominal pain.

WARNING

You should call your doctor immediately if you develop any side effect while taking a drug. If you do develop side-effects it is vitally important that you speak to your doctor before you stop taking your pills. Remember that this list of side-effects isn't complete – you can develop virtually any side effect with virtually any drug – and remember too that some of these side-effects are quite uncommon and many patients can take a drug without getting any side-effects. Always follow your doctor's advice about how and when to take a drug – and if you are in any doubt at all then ask for a second opinion. The fact that one drug may be accompanied by a long list of possible side-effects does not mean that it is necessarily more or less dangerous or more or less likely to produce problems than a drug which has a shorter list of possible side-effects.

CAPTOPRIL

POSSIBLE REASONS TO TAKE IT MAY INCLUDE: For the treatment of mild to moderate hypertension and congestive heart failure and following myocardial infarction.

HOW IS IT PRESCRIBED: Usually twice or three times a day.

POSSIBLE SIDE-EFFECTS MAY INCLUDE: Angioedema involving the extremities, face lips, mucous membranes, tongue, glottis or larynx; neutropenia, anaemia and thrombocytopenia; proteinuria, elevated blood urea and creatinine, elevated serum potassium and acidosis, hypotension and tachycardia. Skin rashes, usually pruritic, may occur – these are usually mild, maculopapular, rarely urticarial and disappear within a few days of dosage reduction, short-term treatment with an antihistamine and/or discontinuing therapy. In a few cases the rash has been associated with fever. Pruritus, flushing, vesicular or bullous rash, photosensitivity; self-limiting taste impairment, weight loss may be associated with the loss of taste; stomatitis, resembling aphthous ulcers; elevation of liver enzymes; gastric irritation, abdominal pain.

WARNING
You should call your doctor immediately if you develop any side effect while taking a drug. If you do develop side-effects it is vitally important that you speak to your doctor before you stop taking your pills. Remember that this list of side-effects isn't complete – you can develop virtually any side effect with virtually any drug – and remember too that some of these side-effects are quite uncommon and many patients can take a drug without getting any side-effects. Always follow your doctor's advice about how and when to take a drug – and if you are in any doubt at all then ask for a second opinion. The fact that one drug may be accompanied by a long list of possible side-effects does not mean that it is necessarily more or less dangerous or more or less likely to produce problems than a drug which has a shorter list of possible side-effects.

CARACE

POSSIBLE REASONS TO TAKE IT MAY INCLUDE: For the treatment of high blood pressure (hypertension) and heart failure.

HOW IS IT PRESCRIBED: Usually once a day; the dosage depends upon the patient's condition and symptoms.

POSSIBLE SIDE-EFFECTS MAY INCLUDE: Hypotension; angioneurotic oedema of the face, extremities, lips, tongue, glottis and/or larynx; dizziness, headache, diarrhoea, fatigue, cough and nausea; rash, and asthenia; myocardial infarction or cerebrovascular accident possibly secondary to excessive hypotension in high-risk patients, palpitation, tachycardia, pancreatitis, abdominal pain, dry mouth, hepatitis (hepatocellular or cholestatic), mood alterations, mental confusion, urticaria, diaphoresis, uraemia, oliguria/anuria, renal dysfunction, acute renal failure, impotence; haemolytic anaemia; symptom complex which may include fever, vasculitis, myalgia arthralgia/arthritis, a positive ANA, elevated erythrocyte sedimentation rate, eosinophilia, and leucocytosis; photosensitivity.

CARBAMAZEPINE

POSSIBLE REASONS TO TAKE IT MAY INCLUDE: For the treatment of epilepsy and the pain of trigeminal neuralgia.

HOW IS IT PRESCRIBED: Usually two or three times a day.

POSSIBLE SIDE-EFFECTS MAY INCLUDE: Dizziness, ataxia, drowsiness, fatigue, headache, blurred vision, depression, hallucinations, appetite loss, agitation, confusion, allergic skin reactions, leucopenia, nausea, vomiting.

WARNING

You should call your doctor immediately if you develop any side effect while taking a drug. If you do develop side-effects it is vitally important that you speak to your doctor before you stop taking your pills. Remember that this list of side-effects isn't complete – you can develop virtually any side effect with virtually any drug – and remember too that some of these side-effects are quite uncommon and many patients can take a drug without getting any side-effects. Always follow your doctor's advice about how and when to take a drug – and if you are in any doubt at all then ask for a second opinion. The fact that one drug may be accompanied by a long list of possible side-effects does not mean that it is necessarily more or less dangerous or more or less likely to produce problems than a drug which has a shorter list of possible side-effects.

CARDURA

POSSIBLE REASONS TO TAKE IT MAY INCLUDE: For the treatment of high blood pressure.

HOW IS IT PRESCRIBED: Once a day.

POSSIBLE SIDE-EFFECTS MAY INCLUDE: Dizziness, vertigo, fatigue, headache, asthenia and oedema.

CAVED-S

POSSIBLE REASONS TO TAKE IT MAY INCLUDE: For the treatment of peptic ulcer.

HOW IS IT PRESCRIBED: The tablets should be taken between meals.

POSSIBLE SIDE-EFFECTS MAY INCLUDE: Mild diarrhoea; effects of acute bismuth intoxication, as observed after intramuscular injection of bismuth salts, include gastro-intestinal disturbances, anorexia, headache, malaise, skin reactions, discolourations of mucous membranes, mild jaundice; if albuminuria or stomatitis occurs, therapy should be immediately withdrawn as serious ulceration stomatitis or renal failure may result. A reversible neurological syndrome, characterised by deterioration of mental ability, confusion, tremor and impaired co-ordination has occurred in colostomy and ileostomy patients after long-term oral intake of more than 5 gm per day of bismuth salts. Intestinal bacteria may reduce bismuth subnitrate to nitrite, causing nitrite poisoning with sufficiently large doses.

CEPOREX

POSSIBLE REASONS TO TAKE IT MAY INCLUDE: For the treatment of the following conditions when caused by susceptible bacteria: respiratory tract infections; ear, nose and throat infections; urinary tract infections; gynaecological and obstetric infections; skin, soft-tissue and bone infections; gonorrhoea and dental infections. As prophylaxis treatment for patients with heart disease undergoing dental treatment as an alternative to penicillin.

HOW IS IT PRESCRIBED: Available as tablets, capsules, syrup and paediatric drops. Usually, for most infections: 1 g twice a day.

POSSIBLE SIDE-EFFECTS MAY INCLUDE: Gastro-intestinal disturbances such as nausea, vomiting and diarrhoea; pseudomembranous colitis; prolonged use may lead to overgrowth of non-susceptible organisms, e.g., candida which may present as vulvo-vaginitis; reversible neutropenia, drug rashes both urticarial and maculopapular; severe skin reactions, toxic epidermal necrolysis (exanthematic necrolysis), and hypersensitivity reactions including angioedema and anaphylaxis; reversible interstitial nephritis.

CHLOROMYCETIN
OPHTHALMIC

POSSIBLE REASONS TO TAKE IT MAY INCLUDE: For the treatment of bacterial conjunctivitis.

HOW IS IT PRESCRIBED: Usually two drops or a small amount of the ointment applied to the affected eye every three hours, or more frequently if required. Treatment should be continued for at least 48 hours after the eye appears normal.

POSSIBLE SIDE-EFFECTS MAY INCLUDE: Bone-marrow hypoplasia, including aplastic anaemia.

CHLORPROMAZINE

POSSIBLE REASONS TO TAKE IT MAY INCLUDE: For the treatment of violent behaviour, nausea and vomiting of terminal illness, schizophrenia, hiccups.

HOW IS IT PRESCRIBED: Usually three a day.

POSSIBLE SIDE-EFFECTS MAY INCLUDE: Liver problems, hypotension, heart problems, blood problems, tremor and other symptoms of Parkinsonism, rashes, sensitivity to sunlight.

CIMETIDINE

POSSIBLE REASONS TO TAKE IT MAY INCLUDE: For the treatment of ulcers in the stomach and duodenum.

HOW IS IT PRESCRIBED: Usually once or twice a day for at least a month.

POSSIBLE SIDE-EFFECTS MAY INCLUDE: Diarrhoea, dizziness, rash, tiredness, swollen breasts in men, liver damage.

WARNING

You should call your doctor immediately if you develop any side effect while taking a drug. If you do develop side-effects it is vitally important that you speak to your doctor before you stop taking your pills. Remember that this list of side-effects isn't complete – you can develop virtually any side effect with virtually any drug – and remember too that some of these side-effects are quite uncommon and many patients can take a drug without getting any side-effects. Always follow your doctor's advice about how and when to take a drug – and if you are in any doubt at all then ask for a second opinion. The fact that one drug may be accompanied by a long list of possible side-effects does not mean that it is necessarily more or less dangerous or more or less likely to produce problems than a drug which has a shorter list of possible side-effects.

CIPROFLOXACIN

POSSIBLE REASONS TO TAKE IT MAY INCLUDE: For the treatment of infections.

HOW IS IT PRESCRIBED: Usually twice a day.

POSSIBLE SIDE-EFFECTS MAY INCLUDE: Nausea, diarrhoea, vomiting, dyspepsia, abdominal pain, headache, restlessness, rash, dizziness, pruritis, convulsions, confusion, hallucinations, liver problems, kidney problems.

CIPROXIN

POSSIBLE REASONS TO TAKE IT MAY INCLUDE: For the treatment of infections.

HOW IS IT PRESCRIBED: Usually twice a day.

POSSIBLE SIDE-EFFECTS MAY INCLUDE: Nausea, diarrhoea, vomiting, dyspepsia, abdominal pain, headache, restlessness, rash, dizziness, pruritis, convulsions, confusion, hallucinations, liver problems, kidney problems.

CISAPRIDE

POSSIBLE REASONS TO TAKE IT MAY INCLUDE: For the treatment of dyspepsia, bloating, heartburn, etc.

HOW IS IT PRESCRIBED: Usually three times a day.

POSSIBLE SIDE-EFFECTS MAY INCLUDE: Abdominal cramps, diarrhoea, headaches, lightheadedness.

CLINORIL

POSSIBLE REASONS TO TAKE IT MAY INCLUDE: For the treatment of arthritis.

HOW IS IT PRESCRIBED: Usually twice a day.

POSSIBLE SIDE-EFFECTS MAY INCLUDE: Gastro-intestinal pain, dyspepsia, nausea, vomiting, diarrhoea, constipation, flatulence, anorexia, dizziness, headache, nervousness, tinnitus, rash, vertigo, insomnia, sweating, convulsions, depression, psychosis, aseptic meningitis, blood problems, liver problems, kidney problems, heart problems, visual disturbances, decreased hearing, metallic or bitter taste.

WARNING

You should call your doctor immediately if you develop any side effect while taking a drug. If you do develop side-effects it is vitally important that you speak to your doctor before you stop taking your pills. Remember that this list of side-effects isn't complete – you can develop virtually any side effect with virtually any drug – and remember too that some of these side-effects are quite uncommon and many patients can take a drug without getting any side-effects. Always follow your doctor's advice about how and when to take a drug – and if you are in any doubt at all then ask for a second opinion. The fact that one drug may be accompanied by a long list of possible side-effects does not mean that it is necessarily more or less dangerous or more or less likely to produce problems than a drug which has a shorter list of possible side-effects.

CLOMID

POSSIBLE REASONS TO TAKE IT MAY INCLUDE: For the treatment of infertility.

HOW IS IT PRESCRIBED: Usually once a day.

POSSIBLE SIDE-EFFECTS MAY INCLUDE: Ovarian enlargement, vasomotor flushes, abdominal-pelvic discomfort, nausea and vomiting, breast discomfort, visual symptoms, headache, intermenstrual spotting or menorrhagia

---

WARNING

You should call your doctor immediately if you develop any side effect while taking a drug. If you do develop side-effects it is vitally important that you speak to your doctor before you stop taking your pills. Remember that this list of side-effects isn't complete – you can develop virtually any side effect with virtually any drug – and remember too that some of these side-effects are quite uncommon and many patients can take a drug without getting any side-effects. Always follow your doctor's advice about how and when to take a drug – and if you are in any doubt at all then ask for a second opinion. The fact that one drug may be accompanied by a long list of possible side-effects does not mean that it is necessarily more or less dangerous or more or less likely to produce problems than a drug which has a shorter list of possible side-effects.

CLOMIPHENE

POSSIBLE REASONS TO TAKE IT MAY INCLUDE: For the treatment of infertility.

HOW IS IT PRESCRIBED: Usually once a day.

POSSIBLE SIDE-EFFECTS MAY INCLUDE: Ovarian enlargement, vasomotor flushes, abdominal-pelvic discomfort, nausea and vomiting, breast discomfort, visual symptoms, headache, intermenstrual spotting or menorrhagia

---

WARNING

You should call your doctor immediately if you develop any side effect while taking a drug. If you do develop side-effects it is vitally important that you speak to your doctor before you stop taking your pills. Remember that this list of side-effects isn't complete – you can develop virtually any side effect with virtually any drug – and remember too that some of these side-effects are quite uncommon and many patients can take a drug without getting any side-effects. Always follow your doctor's advice about how and when to take a drug – and if you are in any doubt at all then ask for a second opinion. The fact that one drug may be accompanied by a long list of possible side-effects does not mean that it is necessarily more or less dangerous or more or less likely to produce problems than a drug which has a shorter list of possible side-effects.

CO-DYDRAMOL

POSSIBLE REASONS TO TAKE IT MAY INCLUDE: For the treatment of mild to moderate pain.

HOW IS IT PRESCRIBED: One to two tablets every four to six hours as required. The maximum should be eight tablets daily.

POSSIBLE SIDE-EFFECTS MAY INCLUDE: Constipation, nausea and headache.

CO-PROXAMOL

POSSIBLE REASONS TO TAKE IT MAY INCLUDE: For the management of mild to moderate pain.

HOW IS IT PRESCRIBED: Usually two tablets three or four times daily. Patients should not normally exceed the recommended dose. Fatalities within the first hour of overdosage are not uncommon and can occur within 15 minutes. Some deaths have occurred as a consequence of the accidental ingestion of excessive quantities of this drug alone, or in combination with other drugs.

POSSIBLE SIDE-EFFECTS MAY INCLUDE: Dizziness, sedation, nausea and vomiting; constipation, abdominal pain, rashes, light-headedness, headache, weakness, euphoria, dysphoria, hallucinations and minor visual disturbances. Co-proxamol is not suitable for patients who are suicidal or addiction-prone. When taken in higher than recommended doses over long periods of time the drug can produce drug dependence.

COLPERMIN

POSSIBLE REASONS TO TAKE IT MAY INCLUDE: For the treatment of symptoms of discomfort and of abdominal colic and distension experienced by patients with irritable bowel syndrome. Also for the treatment of intestinal spasm secondary to other gastro-intestinal disorders, e.g. diverticular disease.

HOW IS IT PRESCRIBED: Usually one capsule three times a day, taken 30-60 minutes before food with a small quantity of water. The capsules should not be taken immediately after food. The dose may be increased to two capsules, three times a day when discomfort is more severe. The capsules should be taken until symptoms resolve, usually within one or two weeks. At times when symptoms are more persistent, the capsules can be continued for longer periods of between two to three months.

POSSIBLE SIDE-EFFECTS MAY INCLUDE: Occasional heartburn, perianal irritation; allergic reactions to menthol, which include erythematous skin rash, headache, bradycardia, muscle tremor and ataxia.

CORACTEN

POSSIBLE REASONS TO TAKE IT MAY INCLUDE: For the treatment of heart pain and high blood pressure.

HOW IS IT PRESCRIBED: To be taken orally with a little fluid

POSSIBLE SIDE-EFFECTS MAY INCLUDE: Headache, dizziness, flushing, nausea, lethargy, increased frequency of passing urine, dyspepsia, heartburn, palpitation, eye pain, depression.

CORDILOX

POSSIBLE REASONS TO TAKE IT MAY INCLUDE: For the treatment of heart problems and high blood pressure.

HOW IS IT PRESCRIBED: Usually two or three times a day.

POSSIBLE SIDE-EFFECTS MAY INCLUDE: Constipation, flushing, headaches, nausea, vomiting.

WARNING

You should call your doctor immediately if you develop any side effect while taking a drug. If you do develop side-effects it is vitally important that you speak to your doctor before you stop taking your pills. Remember that this list of side-effects isn't complete – you can develop virtually any side effect with virtually any drug – and remember too that some of these side-effects are quite uncommon and many patients can take a drug without getting any side-effects. Always follow your doctor's advice about how and when to take a drug – and if you are in any doubt at all then ask for a second opinion. The fact that one drug may be accompanied by a long list of possible side-effects does not mean that it is necessarily more or less dangerous or more or less likely to produce problems than a drug which has a shorter list of possible side-effects.

CYTOTEC

POSSIBLE REASONS TO TAKE IT MAY INCLUDE: For healing of ulcers, including those caused by anti-arthritis drugs.

HOW IS IT PRESCRIBED: Usually two, three or four times a day.

POSSIBLE SIDE-EFFECTS MAY INCLUDE: Diarrhoea, abdominal pain, dyspepsia, flatulence, nausea and vomiting, menorrhagia, vaginal bleeding and intermenstrual bleeding, skin rashes, dizziness.

DAKTACORT

POSSIBLE REASONS TO TAKE IT MAY INCLUDE: For the topical treatment of inflamed dermatoses where infection by susceptible organisms and inflammation coexist e.g. intertrigo and infected eczema. For moist or dry eczema or dermatitis including atopic eczema, primary irritant or contact allergic eczema or seborrhoeic eczema including that associated with acne. Also for intertriginous eczema including inframammary intertrigo, perianal and genital dermatitis.

HOW IS IT PRESCRIBED: The cream or ointment should usually be applied topically to the affected area two or three times daily.

POSSIBLE SIDE-EFFECTS MAY INCLUDE: Local sensitivity reactions.

WARNING

You should call your doctor immediately if you develop any side effect while taking a drug. If you do develop side-effects it is vitally important that you speak to your doctor before you stop taking your pills. Remember that this list of side-effects isn't complete – you can develop virtually any side effect with virtually any drug – and remember too that some of these side-effects are quite uncommon and many patients can take a drug without getting any side-effects. Always follow your doctor's advice about how and when to take a drug – and if you are in any doubt at all then ask for a second opinion. The fact that one drug may be accompanied by a long list of possible side-effects does not mean that it is necessarily more or less dangerous or more or less likely to produce problems than a drug which has a shorter list of possible side-effects.

DAONIL

POSSIBLE REASONS TO TAKE IT MAY INCLUDE: For the oral treatment of patients with non-insulin dependent diabetes who respond inadequately to dietary measure alone.

HOW IS IT PRESCRIBED: Usually with treatment of previously un-treated diabetics stabilisation can be started with one 5 mg tablet of Daonil daily. The dose should be taken by mouth, with or immediately after breakfast or the first main meal. Where control is satisfactory, one tablet is continued as the maintenance dose. If control is unsatisfactory, the dose can be adjusted.

POSSIBLE SIDE-EFFECTS MAY INCLUDE: Mild gastro-intestinal or allergic skin reactions; cross sensitivity to sulphonamides or their derivatives may occur; transient visual disturbances may occur at the start of treatment; reversible leucopenia and thrombocytopenia; agranulocytosis, pancytopenia and haemolytic anaemia; disturbances of liver function and cholestatic jaundice. Hypoglycaemic symptoms have occasionally been reported when the dose has been administered without due regard to the patient's dietary habits.

DEXFENFLURAMINE

POSSIBLE REASONS TO TAKE IT MAY INCLUDE: To help weight loss in severe obesity.

HOW IS IT PRESCRIBED: Usually twice a day.

POSSIBLE SIDE-EFFECTS MAY INCLUDE: Dry mouth, nausea, constipation, diarrhoea, drowsiness, dizziness, urinary frequency, headache, mood disturbances, weakness, insomnia, symptoms of depression, nervousness and conjunctivitis.

WARNING

You should call your doctor immediately if you develop any side effect while taking a drug. If you do develop side-effects it is vitally important that you speak to your doctor before you stop taking your pills. Remember that this list of side-effects isn't complete – you can develop virtually any side effect with virtually any drug – and remember too that some of these side-effects are quite uncommon and many patients can take a drug without getting any side-effects. Always follow your doctor's advice about how and when to take a drug – and if you are in any doubt at all then ask for a second opinion. The fact that one drug may be accompanied by a long list of possible side-effects does not mean that it is necessarily more or less dangerous or more or less likely to produce problems than a drug which has a shorter list of possible side-effects.

DHC CONTINUS TABLETS

POSSIBLE REASONS TO TAKE IT MAY INCLUDE: For the treatment of chronic severe pain.

HOW IS IT PRESCRIBED: Depending on the strength of the tablet, one or two tablets, 12-hourly.

POSSIBLE SIDE-EFFECTS MAY INCLUDE: Constipation, nausea, vomiting, headache, vertigo and urinary retention.

DIAMICRON

POSSIBLE REASONS TO TAKE IT MAY INCLUDE: For the treatment of maturity onset diabetes mellitus.

HOW IS IT PRESCRIBED: The dose should be adjusted according to the individual patient's response, commencing with one half to one tablet and increasing until adequate control is achieved.

POSSIBLE SIDE-EFFECTS MAY INCLUDE: Hypoglycaemia; abnormalities of hepatic function, hepatic failure, hepatitis, and jaundice; nausea, dyspepsia, diarrhoea and constipation (this type of adverse reaction can be avoided if Diamicron is taken during a meal); skin reactions including rash, pruritus, erythema, bullous eruption; blood dyscrasia including anaemia, leucopenia, thrombocytopenia and granulocytopenia.

DIAZEPAM

POSSIBLE REASONS TO TAKE IT MAY INCLUDE: Commonly used in the short-term (two-four weeks) symptomatic treatment of anxiety that is severe, disabling or subjecting the individual to unacceptable distress, occurring alone or in association with insomnia or short-term psychosomatic, organic or psychotic illness. And short-term (two-four weeks) treatment of conditions where anxiety may be a precipitating or aggravating factor, e.g. tension headaches or migraine attacks.

HOW IS IT PRESCRIBED: The usual dose is 2 mg three times daily. The maximum dose is up to 30 mg daily in divided doses. For insomnia associated with anxiety, 5 mg to 15 mg before retiring. The lowest dose which can control symptoms should be used. Treatment should not be continued at the full dose beyond four weeks. Long-term chronic use is not recommended. Treatment should always be tapered off gradually. Patients who have taken benzodiazepines for a prolonged time may require a longer period during which doses are reduced. Specialist help may be appropriate. When given to elderly or debilitated patients doses should not exceed half those normally recommended.

POSSIBLE SIDE-EFFECTS MAY INCLUDE: Like all medicaments of this type, diazepam may modify patients' performance at skilled tasks (driving, operating machinery, etc.) to a varying degree depending on dosage, administration and individual susceptibility; alcohol may intensify any impairment and should, therefore, be avoided during treatment; diazepam should not be used alone to treat depression or anxiety

---

WARNING
You should call your doctor immediately if you develop any side effect while taking a drug. If you do develop side-effects it is vitally important that you speak to your doctor before you stop taking your pills. Remember that this list of side-effects isn't complete – you can develop virtually any side effect with virtually any drug – and remember too that some of these side-effects are quite uncommon and many patients can take a drug without getting any side-effects. Always follow your doctor's advice about how and when to take a drug – and if you are in any doubt at all then ask for a second opinion. The fact that one drug may be accompanied by a long list of possible side-effects does not mean that it is necessarily more or less dangerous than a drug which has a shorter list of possible side-effects.

associated with depression, since suicide may be precipitated in such patients. Amnesia may occur. In cases of bereavement, psychological adjustments may be inhibited by benzodiazepines. The dependence potential of the benzodiazepines increases when high doses are used, especially when given over long periods. This is particularly so in patients with a history of alcoholism or drug abuse, or in patients with marked personality disorders. Treatment should be withdrawn gradually. Symptoms such as depression, nervousness, rebound insomnia, irritability, sweating, and diarrhoea have been reported following abrupt cessation of treatment in patients receiving even normal therapeutic doses for short periods of time. Withdrawal following excessive dosages may produce confusional states, psychotic manifestations and convulsions. Abnormal psychological reactions to benzodiazepines have been reported. Behavioural effects include paradoxical aggressive outbursts, excitement, confusion, and the uncovering of depression with suicidal tendencies. Extreme caution should therefore be used in prescribing benzodiazepines to patients with personality disorders. In patients with myasthenia gravis, who are prescribed diazepam, care should be taken on account of pre-existing muscle weakness. Common adverse effects include drowsiness, sedation, unsteadiness and ataxia, these are dose related and may persist into the following day, even after a single dose. Other adverse effects include headache, vertigo, hypotension, gastrointestinal upsets, skin rashes, visual disturbances, changes in libido, urinary retention; blood dyscrasias and jaundice. Little is known regarding the efficacy or safety of benzodiazepines in long-term use.

DICLOFENAC

POSSIBLE REASONS TO TAKE IT MAY INCLUDE: For the treatment of all grades of pain and inflammation in a wide range of conditions, including: arthritic conditions: rheumatoid arthritis, osteoarthritis, ankylosing spondylitis, acute gout; acute musculo-skeletal disorders such as periarthritis (e.g. frozen shoulder), tendinitis, tenosynovitis, bursitis; other painful conditions resulting from trauma, including fracture, low back pain, sprains, strains, dislocations, orthopaedic, dental and other minor surgery.

HOW IS IT PRESCRIBED: More suitable for short-term use in acute conditions for which treatment is required for no more than three months. There is no information on the use of diclofenac for more than three months. Usually taken two or three times a day.

POSSIBLE SIDE-EFFECTS MAY INCLUDE: Epigastric pain, other gastro-intestinal disorders (e.g. nausea, vomiting, diarrhoea, abdominal cramps, dyspepsia, flatulence, anorexia); gastro-intestinal bleeding, peptic ulcer (with or without bleeding or perforation), bloody diarrhoea; lower gut disorders (e.g. non-specific haemorrhagic colitis and exacerbations of ulcerative colitis or crohn's proctocolitis), pancreatitis, aphthous stomatitis, glossitis, oesophageal lesions, constipation; headache, dizziness, or vertigo; drowsiness, tiredness; disturbances of sensation, paraesthesia, memory disturbance, disorientation, disturbance of vision (blurred vision, diplopia), impaired hearing, tinnitus, insomnia,

---

WARNING
You should call your doctor immediately if you develop any side effect while taking a drug. If you do develop side-effects it is vitally important that you speak to your doctor before you stop taking your pills. Remember that this list of side-effects isn't complete – you can develop virtually any side effect with virtually any drug – and remember too that some of these side-effects are quite uncommon and many patients can take a drug without getting any side-effects. Always follow your doctor's advice about how and when to take a drug – and if you are in any doubt at all then ask for a second opinion. The fact that one drug may be accompanied by a long list of possible side-effects does not mean that it is necessarily more or less dangerous or more or less likely to produce problems than a drug which has a shorter list of possible side-effects.

irritability, convulsions, depression, anxiety, nightmares, tremor, psychotic reactions; taste alteration disorders; rashes or skin eruptions, urticaria; bullous eruptions, eczema, erythema multiforme, Stevens-Johnson Syndrome, Lyell's Syndrome, (acute toxic epidermolysis), erythroderma (exfoliative dermatitis), loss of hair, photosensitivity reactions, purpura including allergic purpura; acute renal insufficiency, urinary abnormalities (e.g. haematuria, proteinuria), interstitial nephritis, nephrotic syndrome, papillary necrosis; liver problems including hepatitis (in isolated cases fulminant) with or without jaundice; thrombocytopenia, leucopenia, agranulocytosis, haemolytic anaemia, aplastic anaemia; oedema, hypersensitivity reactions (e.g. bronchospasm, anaphylactic/anaphylactoid systemic reactions including hypotension); impotence, palpitation, chest pain, hypertension.

DIFLUNISAL

POSSIBLE REASONS TO TAKE IT MAY INCLUDE: For the treatment of pain.

HOW IS IT PRESCRIBED: Usually two or three times a day

POSSIBLE SIDE-EFFECTS MAY INCLUDE: Gastro-intestinal pain, dyspepsia, diarrhoea, nausea, rash, headache, vomiting, constipation, flatulence, dizziness, somnolence, insomnia, tinnitus, fatigue, peptic ulcer, gastro-intestinal bleeding, anorexia, jaundice, liver problems, gastritis, pruritus, sweating, kidney problems, vertigo, lightheadedness, nervousness, depression, hallucinations, confusion, blood problems, blurred vision.

DIGOXIN

POSSIBLE REASONS TO TAKE IT MAY INCLUDE: For the treatment of heart failure.

HOW IS IT PRESCRIBED: Dosage tailored for each patient's needs.

POSSIBLE SIDE-EFFECTS MAY INCLUDE: Anorexia, nausea, vomiting, diarrhoea, breast enlargement in men, weakness, apathy, fatigue, malaise, headache, visual disturbances, depression, psychosis, skin rashes, heart irregularities.

WARNING

You should call your doctor immediately if you develop any side effect while taking a drug. If you do develop side-effects it is vitally important that you speak to your doctor before you stop taking your pills. Remember that this list of side-effects isn't complete – you can develop virtually any side effect with virtually any drug – and remember too that some of these side-effects are quite uncommon and many patients can take a drug without getting any side-effects. Always follow your doctor's advice about how and when to take a drug – and if you are in any doubt at all then ask for a second opinion. The fact that one drug may be accompanied by a long list of possible side-effects does not mean that it is necessarily more or less dangerous or more or less likely to produce problems than a drug which has a shorter list of possible side-effects.

DILTIAZEM

POSSIBLE REASONS TO TAKE IT MAY INCLUDE: For the management of angina pectoris.

HOW IS IT PRESCRIBED: Usually three times a day.

POSSIBLE SIDE-EFFECTS MAY INCLUDE: Nausea, headache, skin rashes, oedema of the ankles, flushing, bradycardia.

DILZEM

POSSIBLE REASONS TO TAKE IT MAY INCLUDE: For the management of angina pectoris and treatment of mild to moderate hypertension.

HOW IS IT PRESCRIBED: Usually twice a day.

POSSIBLE SIDE-EFFECTS MAY INCLUDE: Nausea, headache, skin rash, oedema of the legs, flushing; bradycardia; anorexia.

DISTALGESIC

POSSIBLE REASONS TO TAKE IT MAY INCLUDE: For the treatment of mild to moderate pain.

HOW IS IT PRESCRIBED: Usually two tablets three or four times daily. Patients should not normally exceed the recommended dose. Fatalities within the first hour of overdosage are not uncommon and can occur within 15 minutes. Some deaths have occurred as a consequence of the accidental ingestion of excessive quantities of this drug alone, or in combination with other drugs.

POSSIBLE SIDE-EFFECTS MAY INCLUDE: Dizziness, sedation, nausea and vomiting; constipation, abdominal pain, rashes, light-headedness, headache, weakness, euphoria, dysphoria, hallucinations and minor visual disturbances. Distalgesic is not suitable for patients who are suicidal or addiction-prone. When taken in higher than recommended doses over long periods of time the drug can produce drug dependence.

DOLOBID

POSSIBLE REASONS TO TAKE IT MAY INCLUDE: For the treatment of pain.

HOW IS IT PRESCRIBED: Usually two or three times a day

POSSIBLE SIDE-EFFECTS MAY INCLUDE: Gastro-intestinal pain, dyspepsia, diarrhoea, nausea, rash, headache, vomiting, constipation, flatulence, dizziness, somnolence, insomnia, tinnitus, fatigue, peptic ulcer, gastro-intestinal bleeding, anorexia, jaundice, liver problems, gastritis, pruritus, sweating, kidney problems, vertigo, lightheadedness, nervousness, depression, hallucinations, confusion, blood problems, blurred vision.

DOTHIEPIN

POSSIBLE REASONS TO TAKE IT MAY INCLUDE: For the treatment of symptoms of depressive illness, especially where an anti-anxiety effect is required.

HOW IT IS PRESCRIBED: Divided doses or a single dose at night. A daily dose given as a single night-time dose is sometimes more effective and even better tolerated than the conventional divided day-time dosage. There is evidence that this single night-time dose improves the sleep pattern of the depressed patient.

POSSIBLE SIDE-EFFECTS MAY INCLUDE: Atropine-like side-effects including dry mouth, disturbances of accommodation, tachycardia, constipation and hesitancy of micturition; drowsiness, sweating, postural hypotension, tremor and skin rashes; interference with sexual function; depression of the bone marrow, agranulocytosis, hepatitis (including altered liver function), cholestatic jaundice, hypomania and convulsions; psychotic manifestations, including mania and paranoid delusions may be exacerbated during treatment with tricyclic antidepressants. Withdrawal symptoms may occur on abrupt cessation of tricyclic therapy and include insomnia, irritability and excessive perspiration. Similar symptoms in newborn babies whose mothers received tricyclic antidepressants during the third trimester have also been reported. Cardiac arrhythmias and severe hypotension are likely to occur with high dosage or in deliberate overdosage. They may also occur in

---

WARNING

You should call your doctor immediately if you develop any side effect while taking a drug. If you do develop side-effects it is vitally important that you speak to your doctor before you stop taking your pills. Remember that this list of side-effects isn't complete – you can develop virtually any side effect with virtually any drug – and remember too that some of these side-effects are quite uncommon and many patients can take a drug without getting any side-effects. Always follow your doctor's advice about how and when to take a drug – and if you are in any doubt at all then ask for a second opinion. The fact that one drug may be accompanied by a long list of possible side-effects does not mean that it is necessarily more or less dangerous or more or less likely to produce problems than a drug which has a shorter list of possible side-effects.

---

patients with pre-existing heart disease taking normal dosage. Patients likely to drive vehicles or operate machinery should be warned that the drug may impair alertness. It is recommended that antidepressants should be withdrawn gradually. The elderly are particularly likely to experience adverse reactions to antidepressants, especially agitation, confusion and postural hypotension.

DOXAZOSIN

POSSIBLE REASONS TO TAKE IT MAY INCLUDE: For the treatment of high blood pressure.

HOW IS IT PRESCRIBED: Once a day.

POSSIBLE SIDE-EFFECTS MAY INCLUDE: Dizziness, vertigo, fatigue, headache, asthenia and oedema.

DYAZIDE

POSSIBLE REASONS TO TAKE IT MAY INCLUDE: For the treatment of mild to moderate hypertension, alone or in combination with other anti-hypertensive drugs. It is also used to control oedema in cardiac failure, cirrhosis of the liver or the nephrotic syndrome and in that associated with corticosteroid treatment.

HOW IS IT PRESCRIBED: Dependent on the reason its taken. For hypertension: initially one tablet a day after the morning meal, thereafter adjusted to the patient's needs. In oedema: the usual starting dose is one table twice a day after meals. The maintenance dosage is usually one tablet a day.

POSSIBLE SIDE-EFFECTS MAY INCLUDE: Nausea, vomiting, diarrhoea, muscle cramps, weakness, dizziness, headache, dry mouth, thirst, undesirable decreases in blood pressure and rash; photosensitivity; anaphylaxis.

WARNING

You should call your doctor immediately if you develop any side effect while taking a drug. If you do develop side-effects it is vitally important that you speak to your doctor before you stop taking your pills. Remember that this list of side-effects isn't complete – you can develop virtually any side effect with virtually any drug – and remember too that some of these side-effects are quite uncommon and many patients can take a drug without getting any side-effects. Always follow your doctor's advice about how and when to take a drug – and if you are in any doubt at all then ask for a second opinion. The fact that one drug may be accompanied by a long list of possible side-effects does not mean that it is necessarily more or less dangerous or more or less likely to produce problems than a drug which has a shorter list of possible side-effects.

DYSPAMET

POSSIBLE REASONS TO TAKE IT MAY INCLUDE: For the treatment of ulcers in the stomach and duodenum.

HOW IS IT PRESCRIBED: Usually once or twice a day for at least a month.

POSSIBLE SIDE-EFFECTS MAY INCLUDE: Diarrhoea, dizziness, rash, tiredness, swollen breasts in men, liver damage.

WARNING

You should call your doctor immediately if you develop any side effect while taking a drug. If you do develop side-effects it is vitally important that you speak to your doctor before you stop taking your pills. Remember that this list of side-effects isn't complete – you can develop virtually any side effect with virtually any drug – and remember too that some of these side-effects are quite uncommon and many patients can take a drug without getting any side-effects. Always follow your doctor's advice about how and when to take a drug – and if you are in any doubt at all then ask for a second opinion. The fact that one drug may be accompanied by a long list of possible side-effects does not mean that it is necessarily more or less dangerous or more or less likely to produce problems than a drug which has a shorter list of possible side-effects.

ELTROXIN

POSSIBLE REASONS TO TAKE IT MAY INCLUDE: For the treatment of hypothyroidism.

HOW IS IT PRESCRIBED: Dosage tailored for each patient's needs.

POSSIBLE SIDE-EFFECTS MAY INCLUDE: Anginal pain, cardiac arrhythmias, palpitation, and cramps in skeletal muscle; also tachycardia, diarrhoea, vomiting, tremors, restlessness, excitability, insomnia, headache, flushing, sweating, excessive loss of weight and muscular weakness.

ENALAPRIL MALEATE

POSSIBLE REASONS TO TAKE IT MAY INCLUDE: For the treatment of hypertension: all grades of essential hypertension and renovascular hypertension. For the treatment of heart failure. Prevention of symptomatic heart failure. Prevention of coronary ischaemic events in patients with left-ventricular dysfunction.

HOW IS IT PRESCRIBED: Usually once a day.

POSSIBLE SIDE-EFFECTS MAY INCLUDE: Severe hypotension and renal failure; dizziness, headaches; fatigue, asthenia, hypotension, orthostatic hypotension, syncope, nausea, diarrhoea, muscle cramps, rash, cough; renal dysfunction, renal failure, and oliguria.

EQUAGESIC

POSSIBLE REASONS TO TAKE IT MAY INCLUDE: Short-term use as pain-killer and muscle relaxant.

HOW IS IT PRESCRIBED: Three or four times a day.

POSSIBLE SIDE-EFFECTS MAY INCLUDE: Drowsiness, dizziness, nausea, ataxia, vomiting, low blood pressure, paraesthesia, paradoxical excitement, hypersensitivity reactions (skin rashes, shaking, chills, fever), blood disorders. Some dependence if dosage recommendation exceeded – with withdrawal symptoms if drug is suddenly stopped.

ERYTHROCIN

POSSIBLE REASONS TO TAKE IT MAY INCLUDE: For the prophylaxis and treatment of infections caused by erythromycin-sensitive organisms.

HOW IS IT PRESCRIBED: For mild to moderate infections 1–2 g daily in divided doses. For severe infections this may be increased to 4 g daily in divided doses. Tablets should be taken before or with meals. Duration of dosing should be related to the severity and site of infection, but generally lies within the range of 5–14 days.

POSSIBLE SIDE-EFFECTS MAY INCLUDE: Nausea, abdominal discomfort, vomiting and diarrhoea; reversible hearing loss; allergic reactions; anaphylaxis; damage to the blood, kidneys, liver or central nervous system; cardiac arrhythmias.

EURAX-HYDROCORTISONE

POSSIBLE REASONS TO TAKE IT MAY INCLUDE: For the management of eczema and dermatitis of all types.

HOW IS IT PRESCRIBED: Usually a thin layer of the cream should be applied to the affected area two to three times a day. Treatment for adults should be limited to 10–14 days or up to seven days if applied to the face. Use with caution in infants and for not more than seven days.

POSSIBLE SIDE-EFFECTS MAY INCLUDE: A burning sensation at the site of application, itching, contact dermatitis/contact allergy may occur.

WARNING

You should call your doctor immediately if you develop any side effect while taking a drug. If you do develop side-effects it is vitally important that you speak to your doctor before you stop taking your pills. Remember that this list of side-effects isn't complete – you can develop virtually any side effect with virtually any drug – and remember too that some of these side-effects are quite uncommon and many patients can take a drug without getting any side-effects. Always follow your doctor's advice about how and when to take a drug – and if you are in any doubt at all then ask for a second opinion. The fact that one drug may be accompanied by a long list of possible side-effects does not mean that it is necessarily more or less dangerous or more or less likely to produce problems than a drug which has a shorter list of possible side-effects.

FELDENE

POSSIBLE REASONS TO TAKE IT MAY INCLUDE: For the management of a variety of conditions requiring anti-inflammatory and/or analgesic activity, such as rheumatoid arthritis, osteoarthritis, ankylosing spondylitis, acute gout, acute musculoskeletal disorders and juvenile chronic arthritis.

HOW IS IT PRESCRIBED: Available as capsules, dispersible tablets, suppositories and intramuscular injection.

POSSIBLE SIDE-EFFECTS MAY INCLUDE: Stomatitis, anorexia, epigastric distress, nausea, constipation, abdominal discomfort, flatulence, diarrhoea, abdominal pain and indigestion; peptic ulceration, perforation and gastro-intestinal bleeding, in rare cases fatal. Ano-rectal reactions to suppositories have presented as local pain, burning, pruritus, tenesmus. Oedema, mainly of the ankle. Possibility of precipitating congestive cardiac failure in elderly patients or those with compromised cardiac function; dizziness, headache, somnolence, insomnia, depression, nervousness, hallucinations, mood alterations, dream abnormalities, mental confusion, paraesthesias and vertigo; rash and pruritus; onycholysis and alopecia; photosensitivity reactions; toxic epidermal necrolysis (Lyell's Disease) and Stevens-Johnson Syndrome; vesiculo-bullous reactions; hypersensitivity reactions such as anaphylaxis, bronchospasm, urticaria/angioneurotic oedema, vasculitis and serum sickness; anaemia, thrombocytopenia, non-thrombocytopenic purpura (Henoch-Schoenlein), leucopenia and eosinophilia; aplastic anaemia, haemolytic anaemia and epistaxis; severe hepatic reactions, including jaundice and cases of fatal hepatitis; palpitations and dyspnoea; metabolic abnormalities such as hypoglycaemia, hyperglycaemia, weight increase or decrease; swollen eyes, blurred vision and eye irritations; malaise, tinnitus.

FELODIPINE

POSSIBLE REASONS TO TAKE IT MAY INCLUDE: For the management of high blood pressure.

HOW IS IT PRESCRIBED: Once a day.

POSSIBLE SIDE-EFFECTS MAY INCLUDE: Dizziness, fatigue, headache, ankle swelling, flushing, rash, palpitations, gingival enlargement.

FEMODENE

POSSIBLE REASONS TO TAKE IT MAY INCLUDE: Oral contraception.

HOW IS IT PRESCRIBED: For the first treatment cycle: one tablet daily for 21 days, starting on the first day of the menstrual cycle. Each subsequent course is started when seven tablet-free days have followed the previous course.

POSSIBLE SIDE-EFFECTS MAY INCLUDE: Nausea, vomiting, headaches, breast tension, changed bodyweight or libido, depressive moods and chloasma; reduction of menstrual flow; missed menstruation; intermenstrual bleeding.

FENBID SPANSULE

POSSIBLE REASONS TO TAKE IT MAY INCLUDE: For the management of various types of arthritis and for general pain relief.

HOW IS IT PRESCRIBED: Usually two, twice a day.

POSSIBLE SIDE-EFFECTS MAY INCLUDE: Gastro intestinal upset or bleeding, rash, thrombocytopenia.

FERROGRAD

POSSIBLE REASONS TO TAKE IT MAY INCLUDE: For the prevention and treatment of iron-deficiency anaemia.

HOW IS IT PRESCRIBED: One tablet a day before food.

POSSIBLE SIDE-EFFECTS MAY INCLUDE: Nausea, vomiting, abdominal pain or discomfort, diarrhoea and/or constipation

FERROUS SULPHATE

POSSIBLE REASONS TO TAKE IT MAY INCLUDE: For the prevention and treatment of iron-deficiency anaemia.

HOW IS IT PRESCRIBED: One tablet a day before food.

POSSIBLE SIDE-EFFECTS MAY INCLUDE: Nausea, vomiting, abdominal pain or discomfort, diarrhoea and/or constipation.

FLAGYL COMPAK

POSSIBLE REASONS TO TAKE IT MAY INCLUDE: For the management of vaginitis where a mixed trichomonal/candidal infection is diagnosed.

HOW IS IT PRESCRIBED: One tablet to be swallowed whole, with half a glassful of water during or after meals, twice daily for seven days. Concurrently, one vaginal insert to be moistened and introduced high into the vagina night and morning for seven days.

POSSIBLE SIDE-EFFECTS MAY INCLUDE: Unpleasant taste in the mouth, furred tongue, nausea, vomiting, gastro-intestinal disturbance; urticaria and angioedema; anaphylaxis; drowsiness, dizziness, headache, ataxia, skin rashes, pruritis, incoordination of movements, darkening of the urine (due to metronidazole metabolite), myalgia and arthralgia.

FLEXIN CONTINUS

POSSIBLE REASONS TO TAKE IT MAY INCLUDE: For the management of rheumatoid arthritis; osteoarthritis; ankylosing spondylitis; gout; degenerative joint disease of the hip; painful musculoskeletal disorders; low-back pain and any periarticular disorders such as bursitis, tendinitis, synovitis, tenosynovitis and capsulitis. Also indicated in inflammation, in pain and oedema following orthopaedic procedures and treatment of dysmenorrhoea.

HOW IS IT PRESCRIBED: In order to reduce the possibility of gastro-intestinal disturbance, the tablets should always be given with food, milk or an antacid. The usual recommended daily dose is 25–200 mg taken in one or two divided doses depending on patient's needs and response.

POSSIBLE SIDE-EFFECTS MAY INCLUDE: Headache, dizziness and dyspepsia; mental confusion, depression, convulsions, depersonalisation, tinnitus; coma has also been reported; anorexia, nausea, vomiting, epigastric distress, abdominal pain and diarrhoea; ulceration of the oesophagus, stomach or duodenum, which may be accompanied by either haemorrhage or perforation; gastro-intestinal bleeding without obvious ulceration; blood dyscrasias, particularly thrombocytopenia; blurred vision and orbital and peri-orbital pain; corneal deposits and retinal disturbances; oedema and increased blood pressure and haematuria; hypersensitivity reactions including pruritis,

---

WARNING

You should call your doctor immediately if you develop any side effect while taking a drug. If you do develop side-effects it is vitally important that you speak to your doctor before you stop taking your pills. Remember that this list of side-effects isn't complete – you can develop virtually any side effect with virtually any drug – and remember too that some of these side-effects are quite uncommon and many patients can take a drug without getting any side-effects. Always follow your doctor's advice about how and when to take a drug – and if you are in any doubt at all then ask for a second opinion. The fact that one drug may be accompanied by a long list of possible side-effects does not mean that it is necessarily more or less dangerous or more or less likely to produce problems than a drug which has a shorter list of possible side-effects.

urticaria, angiitis, erythema nodosum; hair loss; acute respiratory distress including sudden dyspnoea and asthma; bronchospasm may be precipitated in patients suffering from, or with a previous history of bronchial asthma or allergic disease; nephrotoxocity in various forms, interstitial nephritis, nephrotic syndrome and renal failure.

FLUNITRAZEPAM

POSSIBLE REASONS TO TAKE IT MAY INCLUDE: For the management of insomnia.

HOW IS IT PRESCRIBED: At bedtime. The lowest dose which can control symptoms should be used. Treatment should not be continued at the full dose beyond four weeks. Long-term chronic use is not recommended. Treatment should always be tapered off gradually. Patients who have taken benzodiazepines for a prolonged time may require a longer period during which doses are reduced. Specialist help may be appropriate.

POSSIBLE SIDE-EFFECTS MAY INCLUDE: Drowsiness, confusion, headache, vertigo, hypotension, gastro-intestinal upsets, skin rashes, visual disturbances, changes in libido, urinary retention, blood problems, jaundice. Little is known regarding the efficacy or safety of benzodiazepines in long term use

---

WARNING
You should call your doctor immediately if you develop any side effect while taking a drug. If you do develop side-effects it is vitally important that you speak to your doctor before you stop taking your pills. Remember that this list of side-effects isn't complete – you can develop virtually any side effect with virtually any drug – and remember too that some of these side-effects are quite uncommon and many patients can take a drug without getting any side-effects. Always follow your doctor's advice about how and when to take a drug – and if you are in any doubt at all then ask for a second opinion. The fact that one drug may be accompanied by a long list of possible side-effects does not mean that it is necessarily more or less dangerous or more or less likely to produce problems than a drug which has a shorter list of possible side-effects.

FLUOXETINE HYDROCHLORIDE

POSSIBLE REASONS TO TAKE IT MAY INCLUDE: For the treatment of the symptoms of depressive illness, especially where sedation is not required. It is also used in the treatment of bulimia nervosa.

HOW IS IT PRESCRIBED: For depression in adults a dose of 20 mg/day is recommended. Use in children is not recommended, as safety and efficacy have not been established.

POSSIBLE SIDE-EFFECTS MAY INCLUDE: Angioneurotic oedema, urticaria and other allergic reactions; asthenia, fever, nausea, diarrhoea, dry mouth, appetite loss, dyspepsia, vomiting; abnormal liver function tests; headache, nervousness, insomnia, drowsiness, anxiety, tremor, dizziness, fatigue, decreased libido, seizures; hypomania or mania occurred in approximately one per cent of fluoxetine-treated trial patients; dyskinesia, movement disorders developing in patients with risk factors and worsening of pre-existing movement disorders, neuroleptic malignant syndrome-like events; pharyngitis, dyspnoea; pulmonary events, dyspnoea may be the only preceding symptom; rash and/or urticaria; serious systemic reactions, possibly related to vasculitis, have developed in patients with rash, and death has been reported; excessive sweating, serum sickness and anaphylactoid reactions; hair loss, usually reversible; sexual dysfunction (delayed or inhibited orgasm).

WARNING

You should call your doctor immediately if you develop any side effect while taking a drug. If you do develop side-effects it is vitally important that you speak to your doctor before you stop taking your pills. Remember that this list of side-effects isn't complete – you can develop virtually any side effect with virtually any drug – and remember too that some of these side-effects are quite uncommon and many patients can take a drug without getting any side-effects. Always follow your doctor's advice about how and when to take a drug – and if you are in any doubt at all then ask for a second opinion. The fact that one drug may be accompanied by a long list of possible side-effects does not mean that it is necessarily more or less dangerous or more or less likely to produce problems than a drug which has a shorter list of possible side-effects.

FLURBIPROFEN

POSSIBLE REASONS TO TAKE IT MAY INCLUDE: For the treatment of arthritis, back pain, period pain, migraine, dental pain, strains, sprains and other pains.

HOW IS IT PRESCRIBED: Several times a day.

POSSIBLE SIDE-EFFECTS MAY INCLUDE: Dyspepsia, nausea, vomiting, gastro-intestinal haemorrhage, diarrhoea, mouth ulcers, rashes, jaundice, blood problems, fluid retention and oedema.

FLUVASTATIN

POSSIBLE REASONS TO TAKE IT MAY INCLUDE: To lower blood cholesterol.

HOW IS IT PRESCRIBED: Usually once a day.

POSSIBLE SIDE-EFFECTS MAY INCLUDE: Dyspepsia, abdominal pain, nausea, insomnia, headache.

FLUVIRIN

POSSIBLE REASONS TO TAKE IT MAY INCLUDE: Protection against influenza.

HOW IS IT PRESCRIBED: By deep subcutaneous or intramuscular injection.

POSSIBLE SIDE-EFFECTS MAY INCLUDE: Redness and soreness at the site of the injection; headache, pyrexia and a feeling of malaise.

FOSFOMYCIN

POSSIBLE REASONS TO TAKE IT MAY INCLUDE: For the management of urinary tract infections.

HOW IS IT PRESCRIBED: Once a day.

POSSIBLE SIDE-EFFECTS MAY INCLUDE: Gastro-intestinal disturbances, rash.

FROBEN

POSSIBLE REASONS TO TAKE IT MAY INCLUDE: For the treatment of arthritis, back pain, period pain, migraine, dental pain, strains, sprains and other pains.

HOW IS IT PRESCRIBED: Several times a day.

POSSIBLE SIDE-EFFECTS MAY INCLUDE: Dyspepsia, nausea, vomiting, gastro-intestinal haemorrhage, diarrhoea, mouth ulcers, rashes, jaundice, blood problems, fluid retention and oedema.

FRUMIL

POSSIBLE REASONS TO TAKE IT MAY INCLUDE: For the management of retained fluid/increasing urine flow.

HOW IS IT PRESCRIBED: The tablets should be taken in the morning. The normal adult dose is one tablet although this may be increased to two tablets.

POSSIBLE SIDE-EFFECTS MAY INCLUDE: Malaise, gastric upset, nausea, vomiting, diarrhoea, and constipation; skin rashes, pruritis; minor psychiatric disturbances; disturbances in liver-function tests, ototoxicity; bone marrow depression.

FRUSEMIDE

POSSIBLE REASONS TO TAKE IT MAY INCLUDE: For the management of retained fluid/increasing urine flow..

HOW IS IT PRESCRIBED: Initially once a day.

POSSIBLE SIDE-EFFECTS MAY INCLUDE: Nausea, malaise, gastric upset, headache, low blood pressure, muscle cramps, skin rash.

GAMANIL

POSSIBLE REASONS TO TAKE IT MAY INCLUDE: For the treatment of the symptoms of depressive illness.

HOW IS IT PRESCRIBED: Usually two or three times daily.

POSSIBLE SIDE-EFFECTS MAY INCLUDE: Hypotension, tachycardia; dizziness, drowsiness, agitation, confusion, headache, malaise, paraesthesia and hypomania and convulsions; dryness of mouth, constipation, disturbances of accommodation, urinary hesitancy, urinary retention, sweating, tremor; skin rash, allergic skin reactions; nausea, vomiting. The following side-effects have been found in patients under treatment with tricyclic antidepressants and should therefore be considered as theoretical hazards: psychotic manifestations, including mania and paranoid delusions, may be exacerbated during treatment with tricyclic antidepressants; withdrawal symptoms may occur on abrupt cessation of therapy and include insomnia, irritability and excessive perspiration; adverse effects such as withdrawal symptoms, respiratory depression and agitation have been reported in newborn babies whose mothers have taken tricyclic antidepressants during the last trimester of pregnancy.

GASTROBID CONTINUS

POSSIBLE REASONS TO TAKE IT MAY INCLUDE: For the management of nausea, vomiting, dyspepsia etc.

HOW IS IT PRESCRIBED: Usually twice a day.

POSSIBLE SIDE-EFFECTS MAY INCLUDE: Muscle spasms, drowsiness, diarrhoea, lethargy, dizziness, headache, insomnia, flatulence.

GASTROMAX

POSSIBLE REASONS TO TAKE IT MAY INCLUDE: For the management of nausea, vomiting, dyspepsia etc.

HOW IS IT PRESCRIBED: Usually once a day.

POSSIBLE SIDE-EFFECTS MAY INCLUDE: Muscle spasms, restlessness, fatigue, dizziness.

GLUCOPHAGE

POSSIBLE REASONS TO TAKE IT MAY INCLUDE: For the management of non-insulin-dependent diabetes when diet has failed and especially if the patient is overweight. In insulin-dependent diabetes, Glucophage may be given as an adjuvant to patients whose symptoms are poorly controlled.

HOW IS IT PRESCRIBED: Usually one 850 mg tablet twice a day or one 500 mg tablet three times a day, with or after food. Good diabetic control may be achieved within a few days, but it is not unusual for the full effect to be delayed for up to two weeks.

POSSIBLE SIDE-EFFECTS MAY INCLUDE: Gastro-intestinal disturbances; lactic acidosis (a medical emergency which must be treated in hospital).

WARNING

You should call your doctor immediately if you develop any side effect while taking a drug. If you do develop side-effects it is vitally important that you speak to your doctor before you stop taking your pills. Remember that this list of side-effects isn't complete – you can develop virtually any side effect with virtually any drug – and remember too that some of these side-effects are quite uncommon and many patients can take a drug without getting any side-effects. Always follow your doctor's advice about how and when to take a drug – and if you are in any doubt at all then ask for a second opinion. The fact that one drug may be accompanied by a long list of possible side-effects does not mean that it is necessarily more or less dangerous or more or less likely to produce problems than a drug which has a shorter list of possible side-effects.

GOPTEN

POSSIBLE REASONS TO TAKE IT MAY INCLUDE: For the management of high blood pressure.

HOW IS IT PRESCRIBED: Usually once a day.

POSSIBLE SIDE-EFFECTS MAY INCLUDE: Cough, headache, asthenia, dizziness, rash, hypotension, palpitations, angioneurotic oedema, nausea.

IBUPROFEN

POSSIBLE REASONS TO TAKE IT MAY INCLUDE: For the treatment of arthritis, rheumatoid arthritis, including juvenile rheumatoid arthritis, and soft-tissue injuries such as sprains and strains. Also prescribed for the relief of mild to moderate pain such as dysmenorrhoea, dental and post-operative pain and for the symptomatic relief of headache including migraine headache.

HOW IS IT PRESCRIBED: Recommended dosage for adults is 1200-1800 mg daily in divided doses. Some patients can be maintained on 600-1200 mg daily.

POSSIBLE SIDE-EFFECTS MAY INCLUDE: Nausea, vomiting, diarrhoea, dyspepsia, abdominal pain; skin rashes; thrombocytopenia.

WARNING

You should call your doctor immediately if you develop any side effect while taking a drug. If you do develop side-effects it is vitally important that you speak to your doctor before you stop taking your pills. Remember that this list of side-effects isn't complete – you can develop virtually any side effect with virtually any drug – and remember too that some of these side-effects are quite uncommon and many patients can take a drug without getting any side-effects. Always follow your doctor's advice about how and when to take a drug – and if you are in any doubt at all then ask for a second opinion. The fact that one drug may be accompanied by a long list of possible side-effects does not mean that it is necessarily more or less dangerous or more or less likely to produce problems than a drug which has a shorter list of possible side-effects.

INDERAL

POSSIBLE REASONS TO TAKE IT MAY INCLUDE: For the control of hypertension, the management of angina pectoris, the long-term prophylaxis against reinfarction after recovery from acute myocardial infarction; the control of most forms of cardiac arrythmia; the prophylaxis of migraine; the management of essential tremor, relief of situational anxiety and generalised anxiety symptoms, particularly those of somatic type; prophylaxis of upper gastro-intestinal bleeding in patients with portal hypertension and oesophageal varices; the adjunctive management of thyrotoxicosis and thyrotoxic crisis.

HOW IS IT PRESCRIBED: Usually two, three or four times a day. The dosage depends upon the disorder being treated.

POSSIBLE SIDE-EFFECTS MAY INCLUDE: Bradycardia, heart failure deterioration, postural hypotension which may be associated with syncope, cold extremities; confusion, dizziness, mood changes, nightmares, psychoses and hallucinations, sleep disturbances, hypoglycaemia in children, gastro-intestinal disturbance, purpura, thrombocytopenia, alopecia, dry eyes, psoriasiform skin reactions, exacerbation of psoriasis, skin rashes, paraesthesia; bronchospasm may occur in patients with bronchial asthma or a history of asthmatic complaints, sometimes with fatal outcome; visual disturbances, fatigue and/or lassitude (often transient). Cessation of therapy should be gradual.

WARNING
You should call your doctor immediately if you develop any side effect while taking a drug. If you do develop side-effects it is vitally important that you speak to your doctor before you stop taking your pills. Remember that this list of side-effects isn't complete – you can develop virtually any side effect with virtually any drug – and remember too that some of these side-effects are quite uncommon and many patients can take a drug without getting any side-effects. Always follow your doctor's advice about how and when to take a drug – and if you are in any doubt at all then ask for a second opinion. The fact that one drug may be accompanied by a long list of possible side-effects does not mean that it is necessarily more or less dangerous or more or less likely to produce problems than a drug which has a shorter list of possible side-effects.

INDOCID

POSSIBLE REASONS TO TAKE IT MAY INCLUDE: For the management of arthritis and other sources of pain.

HOW IS IT PRESCRIBED: By mouth or suppository.

POSSIBLE SIDE-EFFECTS MAY INCLUDE: Headaches, dizziness, lightheadedness, depression, vertigo, fatigue, mental confusion, anxiety, syncope, drowsiness, convulsions, coma, peripheral neuropathy, muscle weakness, involuntary muscle movements, insomnia, psychiatric disturbances such as depersonalisation, aggravation of epilepsy and Parkinsonism, nausea, anorexia, vomiting, abdominal pain, constipation, diarrhoea, ulceration of oesophagus, stomach or duodenum (sometimes with bleeding and perforation), stomatitis, gastritis, flatulence, hepatitis, jaundice, increased blood pressure, tachycardia, chest pain, arrhythmia, palpitations, hypotension, congestive heart failure, pruritus, urticaria, skin rash, loss of hair, bronchospasm, blood problems, blurred vision, double vision, tinnitus, hearing disturbance, kidney problems, vaginal bleeding, flushing, sweating, nose bleeding, breast changes including enlargement and tenderness.

INDOMETHACIN

POSSIBLE REASONS TO TAKE IT MAY INCLUDE: For the management of arthritis and other sources of pain.

HOW IS IT PRESCRIBED: By mouth or suppository.

POSSIBLE SIDE-EFFECTS MAY INCLUDE: Headaches, dizziness, lightheadedness, depression, vertigo, fatigue, mental confusion, anxiety, syncope, drowsiness, convulsions, coma, peripheral neuropathy, muscle weakness, involuntary muscle movements, insomnia, psychiatric disturbances such as depersonalisation, aggravation of epilepsy and Parkinsonism, nausea, anorexia, vomiting, abdominal pain, constipation, diarrhoea, ulceration of oesophagus, stomach or duodenum (sometimes with bleeding and perforation), stomatitis, gastritis, flatulence, hepatitis, jaundice, increased blood pressure, tachycardia, chest pain, arrhythmia, palpitations, hypotension, congestive heart failure, pruritus, urticaria, skin rash, loss of hair, bronchospasm, blood problems, blurred vision, double vision, tinnitus, hearing disturbance, kidney problems, vaginal bleeding, flushing, sweating, nose bleeding, breast changes including enlargement and tenderness.

WARNING
You should call your doctor immediately if you develop any side effect while taking a drug. If you do develop side-effects it is vitally important that you speak to your doctor before you stop taking your pills. Remember that this list of side-effects isn't complete – you can develop virtually any side effect with virtually any drug – and remember too that some of these side-effects are quite uncommon and many patients can take a drug without getting any side-effects. Always follow your doctor's advice about how and when to take a drug – and if you are in any doubt at all then ask for a second opinion. The fact that one drug may be accompanied by a long list of possible side-effects does not mean that it is necessarily more or less dangerous or more or less likely to produce problems than a drug which has a shorter list of possible side-effects.

INNOVACE

POSSIBLE REASONS TO TAKE IT MAY INCLUDE: For the treatment of hypertension: all grades of essential hypertension and renovascular hypertension. For the treatment of heart failure. Prevention of symptomatic heart failure. Prevention of coronary ischaemic events in patients with left-ventricular dysfunction.

HOW IS IT PRESCRIBED: Usually once a day.

POSSIBLE SIDE-EFFECTS MAY INCLUDE: Severe hypotension and renal failure; dizziness, headaches; fatigue, asthenia, hypotension, orthostatic hypotension, syncope, nausea, diarrhoea, muscle cramps, rash, cough; renal dysfunction, renal failure, and oliguria.

WARNING

You should call your doctor immediately if you develop any side effect while taking a drug. If you do develop side-effects it is vitally important that you speak to your doctor before you stop taking your pills. Remember that this list of side-effects isn't complete – you can develop virtually any side effect with virtually any drug – and remember too that some of these side-effects are quite uncommon and many patients can take a drug without getting any side-effects. Always follow your doctor's advice about how and when to take a drug – and if you are in any doubt at all then ask for a second opinion. The fact that one drug may be accompanied by a long list of possible side-effects does not mean that it is necessarily more or less dangerous or more or less likely to produce problems than a drug which has a shorter list of possible side-effects.

ISOTRATE

POSSIBLE REASONS TO TAKE IT MAY INCLUDE: For the prophylaxis of angina pectoris.

HOW IS IT PRESCRIBED: Usually one tablet two or three times daily.

POSSIBLE SIDE-EFFECTS MAY INCLUDE: Hypotension, headache, dizziness and nausea.

ISRADIPINE

POSSIBLE REASONS TO TAKE IT MAY INCLUDE: For the treatment of essential hypertension.

HOW IS IT PRESCRIBED: Usually twice a day.

POSSIBLE SIDE-EFFECTS MAY INCLUDE: Dizziness, flushing, headache, palpitations, tachycardia, palpitation, weight gain, fatigue, abdominal discomfort, skin rash.

ISTIN

POSSIBLE REASONS TO TAKE IT MAY INCLUDE: For the management of hypertension and myocardial ischaemia.

HOW IS IT PRESCRIBED: For both hypertension and angina, usually once daily orally.

POSSIBLE SIDE-EFFECTS MAY INCLUDE: Headache, oedema, fatigue, nausea, flushing and dizziness.

KETOPROFEN

POSSIBLE REASONS TO TAKE IT MAY INCLUDE: For the management of rheumatoid arthritis, osteoarthritis, ankylosing spondylitis, acute articular and periarticular disorders, fibrositis, cervical spondylitis, low-back pain, painful musculoskeletal conditions, dysmenorrhoea, acute gout and control of pain and inflammation following orthopaedic surgery.

HOW IS IT PRESCRIBED: Available as capsules and suppositories. Ketoprofen is administered orally and/or rectally; to limit occurrence of gastro-intestinal disturbance, capsules should always be taken with food. Oral dosage is twice daily and should be taken early in the morning and late at night. Rectal dosage is one suppository late at night supplemented as required with the capsules during the daytime.

POSSIBLE SIDE-EFFECTS MAY INCLUDE: Indigestion, dyspepsia, nausea, constipation, diarrhoea, heartburn and various types of abdominal discomfort; headache, dizziness, mild confusion, vertigo, drowsiness, oedema, mood change and insomnia; peptic ulceration, haemorrhage or perforation; thrombocytopenia, hepatic or renal damage, dermatological and photosensitivity reactions, bronchospasm and anaphylaxis.

WARNING

You should call your doctor immediately if you develop any side effect while taking a drug. If you do develop side-effects it is vitally important that you speak to your doctor before you stop taking your pills. Remember that this list of side-effects isn't complete – you can develop virtually any side effect with virtually any drug – and remember too that some of these side-effects are quite uncommon and many patients can take a drug without getting any side-effects. Always follow your doctor's advice about how and when to take a drug – and if you are in any doubt at all then ask for a second opinion. The fact that one drug may be accompanied by a long list of possible side-effects does not mean that it is necessarily more or less dangerous or more or less likely to produce problems than a drug which has a shorter list of possible side-effects.

LABETALOL

POSSIBLE REASONS TO TAKE IT MAY INCLUDE: For the treatment of high blood pressure and heart pain.

HOW IS IT PRESCRIBED: Usually twice a day.

POSSIBLE SIDE-EFFECTS MAY INCLUDE: Headache, tiredness, dizziness, depressed mood, lethargy, nasal congestion, sweating, ankle swelling, tingling sensation in the scalp, acute retention of urine, difficulty in passing urine, ejaculatory failure, epigastric pain, nausea, vomiting, rash, itching, difficulty in breathing, heart block and jaundice.

WARNING
You should call your doctor immediately if you develop any side effect while taking a drug. If you do develop side-effects it is vitally important that you speak to your doctor before you stop taking your pills. Remember that this list of side-effects isn't complete – you can develop virtually any side effect with virtually any drug – and remember too that some of these side-effects are quite uncommon and many patients can take a drug without getting any side-effects. Always follow your doctor's advice about how and when to take a drug – and if you are in any doubt at all then ask for a second opinion. The fact that one drug may be accompanied by a long list of possible side-effects does not mean that it is necessarily more or less dangerous or more or less likely to produce problems than a drug which has a shorter list of possible side-effects.

LACIDIPINE

POSSIBLE REASONS TO TAKE IT MAY INCLUDE: For the treatment of high blood pressure.

HOW IS IT PRESCRIBED: Usually once a day.

POSSIBLE SIDE-EFFECTS MAY INCLUDE: Flushing, dizziness, headache, palpitations, asthenia, rash, chest pain, gastric upset, nausea.

LACTULOSE SOLUTION BP

POSSIBLE REASONS TO TAKE IT MAY INCLUDE: For the management of constipation.

HOW IS IT PRESCRIBED: Initially twice a day.

POSSIBLE SIDE-EFFECTS MAY INCLUDE: Flatulence and diarrhoea

LANOXIN

POSSIBLE REASONS TO TAKE IT MAY INCLUDE: For the management of heart failure.

HOW IS IT PRESCRIBED: Dosage tailored for each patient's needs.

POSSIBLE SIDE-EFFECTS MAY INCLUDE: Anorexia, nausea, vomiting, diarrhoea, breast enlargement in men, weakness, apathy, fatigue, malaise, headache, visual disturbances, depression, psychosis, skin rashes, heart irregularities.

WARNING

You should call your doctor immediately if you develop any side effect while taking a drug. If you do develop side-effects it is vitally important that you speak to your doctor before you stop taking your pills. Remember that this list of side-effects isn't complete – you can develop virtually any side effect with virtually any drug – and remember too that some of these side-effects are quite uncommon and many patients can take a drug without getting any side-effects. Always follow your doctor's advice about how and when to take a drug – and if you are in any doubt at all then ask for a second opinion. The fact that one drug may be accompanied by a long list of possible side-effects does not mean that it is necessarily more or less dangerous or more or less likely to produce problems than a drug which has a shorter list of possible side-effects.

LARGACTIL

POSSIBLE REASONS TO TAKE IT MAY INCLUDE: Many indications including: violent behaviour, nausea and vomiting of terminal illness, schizophrenia, hiccups.

HOW IS IT PRESCRIBED: Usually three times a day.

POSSIBLE SIDE-EFFECTS MAY INCLUDE: Liver problems, hypotension, heart problems, blood problems, tremor and other symptoms of Parkinsonism, rashes, sensitivity to sunlight.

WARNING
You should call your doctor immediately if you develop any side effect while taking a drug. If you do develop side-effects it is vitally important that you speak to your doctor before you stop taking your pills. Remember that this list of side-effects isn't complete – you can develop virtually any side effect with virtually any drug – and remember too that some of these side-effects are quite uncommon and many patients can take a drug without getting any side-effects. Always follow your doctor's advice about how and when to take a drug – and if you are in any doubt at all then ask for a second opinion. The fact that one drug may be accompanied by a long list of possible side-effects does not mean that it is necessarily more or less dangerous or more or less likely to produce problems than a drug which has a shorter list of possible side-effects.

LASIX

POSSIBLE REASONS TO TAKE IT MAY INCLUDE: For the management of retained fluid/increasing urine flow.

HOW IS IT PRESCRIBED: Initially once a day.

POSSIBLE SIDE-EFFECTS MAY INCLUDE: Nausea, malaise, gastric upset, headache, low blood pressure, muscle cramps, skin rash.

LENTIZOL

POSSIBLE REASONS TO TAKE IT MAY INCLUDE: For treatment of symptoms of depressive illness, especially where sedation is required.

HOW IS IT PRESCRIBED: Commonly a single dose at night by mouth. In the elderly (over 65 years) the initial dose should be increased with caution under close supervision. Half the normal maintenance dose may be sufficient to produce a satisfactory clinical response. The elderly are particularly liable to experience adverse reactions, especially agitation, confusion and postural hypotension. As improvement may not occur during the first two to four weeks of treatment, patients should be closely monitored during this period.

POSSIBLE SIDE-EFFECTS MAY INCLUDE: Impaired alertness; cardiac arrhythmias and hypotension; excessive perspiration; dryness of mouth, blurred vision, constipation, tachycardia and urinary retention; postural hypotension, skin rashes; interference with sexual function, nausea, anorexia and dizziness; drowsiness; depression of the bone marrow, including agranulocytosis; hypomania, peripheral neuropathy; paralytic ileus. Withdrawal symptoms may occur on abrupt cessation of therapy and include insomnia, irritability and excessive perspiration.

WARNING
You should call your doctor immediately if you develop any side effect while taking a drug. If you do develop side-effects it is vitally important that you speak to your doctor before you stop taking your pills. Remember that this list of side-effects isn't complete – you can develop virtually any side effect with virtually any drug – and remember too that some of these side-effects are quite uncommon and many patients can take a drug without getting any side-effects. Always follow your doctor's advice about how and when to take a drug – and if you are in any doubt at all then ask for a second opinion. The fact that one drug may be accompanied by a long list of possible side-effects does not mean that it is necessarily more or less dangerous or more or less likely to produce problems than a drug which has a shorter list of possible side-effects.

LESCOL

POSSIBLE REASONS TO TAKE IT MAY INCLUDE: To lower blood cholesterol.

HOW IS IT PRESCRIBED: Usually once a day.

POSSIBLE SIDE-EFFECTS MAY INCLUDE: Dyspepsia, abdominal pain, nausea, insomnia, headache.

LISINOPRIL

POSSIBLE REASONS TO TAKE IT MAY INCLUDE: For the treatment of high blood pressure (hypertension) and heart failure.

HOW IS IT PRESCRIBED: Usually once a day; the dosage depends upon the patient's condition and symptoms.

POSSIBLE SIDE-EFFECTS MAY INCLUDE: Hypotension; angioneurotic oedema of the face, extremities, lips, tongue, glottis and/ or larynx; dizziness, headache, diarrhoea, fatigue, cough and nausea; rash, and asthenia; myocardial infarction or cerebrovascular accident possibly secondary to excessive hypotension in high-risk patients, palpitation, tachycardia, pancreatitis, abdominal pain, dry mouth, hepatitis (hepatocellular or cholestatic), mood alterations, mental confusion, urticaria, diaphoresis, uraemia, oliguria/anuria, renal dysfunction, acute renal failure, impotence; haemolytic anaemia; symptom complex which may include fever, vasculitis, myalgia arthralgia/arthritis, a positive ANA, elevated erythrocyte sedimentation rate, eosinophilia, and leucocytosis; photosensitivity.

WARNING

You should call your doctor immediately if you develop any side effect while taking a drug. If you do develop side-effects it is vitally important that you speak to your doctor before you stop taking your pills. Remember that this list of side-effects isn't complete – you can develop virtually any side effect with virtually any drug – and remember too that some of these side-effects are quite uncommon and many patients can take a drug without getting any side-effects. Always follow your doctor's advice about how and when to take a drug – and if you are in any doubt at all then ask for a second opinion. The fact that one drug may be accompanied by a long list of possible side-effects does not mean that it is necessarily more or less dangerous or more or less likely to produce problems than a drug which has a shorter list of possible side-effects.

LITHIUM CARBONATE

POSSIBLE REASONS TO TAKE IT MAY INCLUDE: For the treatment of mania, hypomania and some depressions.

HOW IS IT PRESCRIBED: Usually once or twice a day.

POSSIBLE SIDE-EFFECTS MAY INCLUDE: Anorexia, diarrhoea, vomiting, muscle weakness, lack of coordination, drowsiness, lethargy, giddiness, tinnitus, blurred vision, tremor, muscle twitching.

LORAZEPAM

POSSIBLE REASONS TO TAKE IT MAY INCLUDE: For the treatment of anxiety; recommended for short-term use of up to 4 weeks.

HOW IS IT PRESCRIBED: For moderate and severe anxiety commonly 1-4 mg daily in divided doses. As with all benzodiazepines long-term use may lead to dependence and withdrawal symptoms in certain patients. All patients taking lorazepam should be carefully monitored and routine repeat prescriptions should be avoided. Treatment in all patients should be withdrawn gradually with careful monitoring and reassessment to minimise possible withdrawal symptoms. Patients who have taken benzodiazepines for a long time may require a longer period during which doses are reduced. The elderly may respond to lower doses and half the normal adult dose or less may be sufficient.

POSSIBLE SIDE-EFFECTS MAY INCLUDE: Daytime drowsiness; confusion, headache, dizziness, nausea, depression, change in appetite and sleep disturbance; blood dyscrasias and abnormal liver function tests; visual disturbances, hypotension, gastro-intestinal disturbances, skin rashes. The use of benzodiazepines may release suicidal tendencies in depressed patients. Lorazepam should not be used alone to treat depression.

WARNING
You should call your doctor immediately if you develop any side effect while taking a drug. If you do develop side-effects it is vitally important that you speak to your doctor before you stop taking your pills. Remember that this list of side-effects isn't complete – you can develop virtually any side effect with virtually any drug – and remember too that some of these side-effects are quite uncommon and many patients can take a drug without getting any side-effects. Always follow your doctor's advice about how and when to take a drug – and if you are in any doubt at all then ask for a second opinion. The fact that one drug may be accompanied by a long list of possible side-effects does not mean that it is necessarily more or less dangerous or more or less likely to produce problems than a drug which has a shorter list of possible side-effects.

LOSEC

POSSIBLE REASONS TO TAKE IT MAY INCLUDE: For the treatment of oesophageal reflux disease. Treatment of duodenal and benign gastric ulcers.

HOW IS IT PRESCRIBED: Usually once a day.

POSSIBLE SIDE-EFFECTS MAY INCLUDE: Skin rash, urticaria and pruritis; photosensitivity, bullous eruption, erythema multiforme, angioedema and alopecia; diarrhoea, headache; constipation, nausea/vomiting, flatulence and abdominal pain; stomatitis and candidiasis; paraesthesia; dizziness, lightheadedness and feeling faint; somnolence, insomnia and vertigo; reversible mental confusion, agitation, depression and hallucinations; arthritic and myalgic symptoms; blurred vision, taste disturbance, peripheral oedema, increased sweating, gynaecomastia, leucopenia, thrombocytopenia, malaise, fever, bronchospasm; encephalopathy in patients with pre-existing severe liver disease, hepatitis with or without jaundice, interstitial nephritis and hepatic failure.

LUSTRAL

POSSIBLE REASONS TO TAKE IT MAY INCLUDE: For the treatment of symptoms of depressive illness.

HOW IS IT PRESCRIBED: Once a day.

POSSIBLE SIDE-EFFECTS MAY INCLUDE: Dry mouth, nausea, diarrhoea, ejaculatory delay, tremor, increased sweating, dyspepsia, insomnia, somnolence.

WARNING

You should call your doctor immediately if you develop any side effect while taking a drug. If you do develop side-effects it is vitally important that you speak to your doctor before you stop taking your pills. Remember that this list of side-effects isn't complete – you can develop virtually any side effect with virtually any drug – and remember too that some of these side-effects are quite uncommon and many patients can take a drug without getting any side-effects. Always follow your doctor's advice about how and when to take a drug – and if you are in any doubt at all then ask for a second opinion. The fact that one drug may be accompanied by a long list of possible side-effects does not mean that it is necessarily more or less dangerous or more or less likely to produce problems than a drug which has a shorter list of possible side-effects.

MANERIX

POSSIBLE REASONS TO TAKE IT MAY INCLUDE: For the treatment of depression.

HOW IS IT PRESCRIBED: Initially twice a day.

POSSIBLE SIDE-EFFECTS MAY INCLUDE: Headache, dizziness, nausea, sleep disturbances.

MAXOLON

POSSIBLE REASONS TO TAKE IT MAY INCLUDE: For the treatment of nausea, vomiting, dyspepsia, etc.

HOW IS IT PRESCRIBED: Usually three times a day.

POSSIBLE SIDE-EFFECTS MAY INCLUDE: Muscle spasms, drowsiness, diarrhoea, restlessness.

WARNING

You should call your doctor immediately if you develop any side effect while taking a drug. If you do develop side-effects it is vitally important that you speak to your doctor before you stop taking your pills. Remember that this list of side-effects isn't complete – you can develop virtually any side effect with virtually any drug – and remember too that some of these side-effects are quite uncommon and many patients can take a drug without getting any side-effects. Always follow your doctor's advice about how and when to take a drug – and if you are in any doubt at all then ask for a second opinion. The fact that one drug may be accompanied by a long list of possible side-effects does not mean that it is necessarily more or less dangerous or more or less likely to produce problems than a drug which has a shorter list of possible side-effects.

MEFENAMIC ACID

POSSIBLE REASONS TO TAKE IT MAY INCLUDE: For the management of pain, heavy menstrual bleeding and painful periods.

HOW IS IT PRESCRIBED: Usually three times a day.

POSSIBLE SIDE-EFFECTS MAY INCLUDE: Diarrhoea; skin rash; gastrointestinal bleeding, ulceration and perforation; kidney problems; blood problems; bronchospasm in patients suffering from, or with a previous history of bronchial asthma or allergic disease; liver problems; nausea, vomiting, abdominal pain, headache, facial oedema, anaphylaxis, drowsiness, dizziness.

MEPTAZINOL

POSSIBLE REASONS TO TAKE IT MAY INCLUDE: For the treatment of pain.

HOW IS IT PRESCRIBED: Usually one tablet every four hours.

POSSIBLE SIDE-EFFECTS MAY INCLUDE: Nausea, dizziness, vomiting, diarrhoea, increased sweating, rash, vertigo, headache, somnolence, dyspepsia, abdominal pain.

MEPTID

POSSIBLE REASONS TO TAKE IT MAY INCLUDE: For the treatment of pain.

HOW IS IT PRESCRIBED: Usually one tablet every four hours.

POSSIBLE SIDE-EFFECTS MAY INCLUDE: Nausea, dizziness, vomiting, diarrhoea, increased sweating, rash, vertigo, headache, somnolence, dyspepsia, abdominal pain.

MINITRAN

POSSIBLE REASONS TO TAKE IT MAY INCLUDE: Prophylaxis of angina pectoris either alone or in combination with other anti-anginal therapy.

HOW IS IT PRESCRIBED: Treatment usually starts with one Minitran 5 patch per day, with upward dosage titration when necessary. Application can either be for a continuous period of 24 hours or intermittently, incorporating a patch-free interval.

POSSIBLE SIDE-EFFECTS MAY INCLUDE: Headache; arterial hypotension (especially postural), tachycardia, fainting, palpitations, hot flushes, dizziness; nausea and vomiting; reddening of the skin with or without itching or a slight erythematous reaction.

MINOXIDIL

POSSIBLE REASONS TO TAKE IT MAY INCLUDE: For the treatment of hair loss.

HOW IS IT PRESCRIBED: Usually applied to the scalp twice a day.

POSSIBLE SIDE-EFFECTS MAY INCLUDE: Irritant dermatitis, allergic contact dermatitis.

MISOPROSTOL

POSSIBLE REASONS TO TAKE IT MAY INCLUDE: For healing of ulcers, including those caused by anti-arthritis drugs.

HOW IS IT PRESCRIBED: Usually two, three or four times a day.

POSSIBLE SIDE-EFFECTS MAY INCLUDE: Diarrhoea, abdominal pain, dyspepsia, flatulence, nausea and vomiting, menorrhagia, vaginal bleeding and intermenstrual bleeding, skin rashes, dizziness.

MOCLOBEMIDE

POSSIBLE REASONS TO TAKE IT MAY INCLUDE: For the treatment of depression.

HOW IS IT PRESCRIBED: Initially twice a day.

POSSIBLE SIDE-EFFECTS MAY INCLUDE: Headache, dizziness, nausea, sleep disturbances.

MODURETIC

POSSIBLE REASONS TO TAKE IT MAY INCLUDE: For hypertension, congestive heart failure, hepatic cirrhosis with ascites and oedema.

HOW IS IT PRESCRIBED: Usually one or two tablets a day to start with.

POSSIBLE SIDE-EFFECTS MAY INCLUDE: Headache, weakness, fatigue, malaise, chest pain, back pain, syncope; arrythmias, tachycardia, digitalis toxicity, orthostatic hypotension, angina pectoris; anorexia, nausea, vomiting, diarrhoea, constipation, abdominal pain, gastro-intestinal bleeding, appetite changes, abdominal fullness, flatulence, thirst, hiccups; elevated plasma potassium levels, electrolyte imbalance, gout, dehydration; rash, pruritis, flushing, diaphoresis; leg ache, muscle cramps, joint pain; dizziness, vertigo, paraesthesiae, stupor; insomnia, nervousness, mental confusion, depression, sleepiness; dyspnoea; bad taste, visual disturbance, nasal congestion; impotence, dysuria, nocturia, incontinence, renal dysfunction including renal failure; neck/shoulder ache, pain in extremities; abnormal liver function, dyspepsia, jaundice; dry mouth, alopecia; tremors, encephalopathy; decreased libido; cough; tinnitus, increased intra-ocular pressure; polyuria, urinary frequency, bladder spasm; anaphylactic reaction, fever; pancreatitis, cramping; glycosuria, hyperglycaemia, hyperuricaemia; photosensitvity, urticaria; restlessness; respiratory distress, pulmonary oedema; transient blurred vision, blood problems.

WARNING

You should call your doctor immediately if you develop any side effect while taking a drug. If you do develop side-effects it is vitally important that you speak to your doctor before you stop taking your pills. Remember that this list of side-effects isn't complete – you can develop virtually any side effect with virtually any drug – and remember too that some of these side-effects are quite uncommon and many patients can take a drug without getting any side-effects. Always follow your doctor's advice about how and when to take a drug – and if you are in any doubt at all then ask for a second opinion. The fact that one drug may be accompanied by a long list of possible side-effects does not mean that it is necessarily more or less dangerous or more or less likely to produce problems than a drug which has a shorter list of possible side-effects.

MOGADON

POSSIBLE REASONS TO TAKE IT MAY INCLUDE: Mogadon is a benzodiazepine with sedative properties. It works in 30 to 60 minutes to produce sleep which lasts for between six and eight hours. The drug is used in the short-term treatment of insomnia when it is severe, disabling or subjecting the individual to unacceptable distress, and where daytime sedation is acceptable.

HOW IS IT PRESCRIBED: To be taken at night. In elderly or debilitated patients dosage should not exceed half doses normally recommended. The dosage should be adjusted on an individual basis. Treatment should, if possible, be intermittent. The lowest dose which can control symptoms should be used and treatment should not be continued at full dose beyond four weeks. Long-term chronic use is not recommended. Treatment should always be tapered off gradually and patients who have taken benzodiazepines for a prolonged time may require a longer period during which doses are reduced. Mogadon should not be used alone to treat depression or anxiety associated with depression, since suicide may be precipitated in such patients. In cases of bereavement, psychological adjustment may be inhibited by benzodiazepines. Like all medicaments of this type, Mogadon may modify patients' performance at skilled tasks (such as driving, operating machinery, etc.) to a varying degree depending upon dosage, administration and individual susceptibility. Alcohol may intensify impairment and should, therefore, be avoided. The dependence potential of the benzodiazepines increases when high doses are used, especially

---

WARNING

You should call your doctor immediately if you develop any side effect while taking a drug. If you do develop side-effects it is vitally important that you speak to your doctor before you stop taking your pills. Remember that this list of side-effects isn't complete – you can develop virtually any side effect with virtually any drug – and remember too that some of these side-effects are quite uncommon and many patients can take a drug without getting any side-effects. Always follow your doctor's advice about how and when to take a drug – and if you are in any doubt at all then ask for a second opinion. The fact that one drug may be accompanied by a long list of possible side-effects does not mean that it is necessarily more or less dangerous than more or less likely to produce problems than a drug which has a shorter list of possible side-effects.

---

when given over long periods. This is particularly so in patients with a history of alcoholism or drug abuse, or in patients with marked personality disorders. Regular monitoring in such patients is essential. Routine repeat prescriptions should be avoided and treatment should be withdrawn gradually. Symptoms such as depression, nervousness, rebound insomnia, irritability, sweating, and diarrhoea may occur if treatment is suddenly stopped in patients receiving even normal doses for short periods of time. Withdrawal following excessive dosages may produce confusional states, psychotic manifestations and convulsions. An underlying cause for insomnia should be sought before a benzodiazepine is used to treat sleeplessness.

POSSIBLE SIDE-EFFECTS MAY INCLUDE: Drowsiness, sedation, unsteadiness and ataxia; headache, vertigo, hypotension, gastro-intestinal upsets, skin rashes, visual disturbances, changes in libido, urinary retention; blood dyscrasias, jaundice; paradoxical aggressive outbursts, excitement, confusion and the uncovering of depression with suicidal tendencies; The elderly are particularly sensitive to the effects of centrally depressant drugs and may experience confusion, especially if organic brain changes are present. Little is known regarding the efficacy or safety of benzodiazepines in long-term use.

WARNING

You should call your doctor immediately if you develop any side effect while taking a drug. If you do develop side-effects it is vitally important that you speak to your doctor before you stop taking your pills. Remember that this list of side-effects isn't complete – you can develop virtually any side effect with virtually any drug – and remember too that some of these side-effects are quite uncommon and many patients can take a drug without getting any side-effects. Always follow your doctor's advice about how and when to take a drug – and if you are in any doubt at all then ask for a second opinion. The fact that one drug may be accompanied by a long list of possible side-effects does not mean that it is necessarily more or less dangerous or more or less likely to produce problems than a drug which has a shorter list of possible side-effects.

MONURIL

POSSIBLE REASONS TO TAKE IT MAY INCLUDE: For the treatment of urinary tract infection.

HOW IS IT PRESCRIBED: Once a day.

POSSIBLE SIDE-EFFECTS MAY INCLUDE: Gastro-intestinal disturbances, rash.

WARNING
You should call your doctor immediately if you develop any side effect while taking a drug. If you do develop side-effects it is vitally important that you speak to your doctor before you stop taking your pills. Remember that this list of side-effects isn't complete – you can develop virtually any side effect with virtually any drug – and remember too that some of these side-effects are quite uncommon and many patients can take a drug without getting any side-effects. Always follow your doctor's advice about how and when to take a drug – and if you are in any doubt at all then ask for a second opinion. The fact that one drug may be accompanied by a long list of possible side-effects does not mean that it is necessarily more or less dangerous or more or less likely to produce problems than a drug which has a shorter list of possible side-effects.

MOTENS

POSSIBLE REASONS TO TAKE IT MAY INCLUDE: For the treatment of high blood pressure.

HOW IS IT PRESCRIBED: Usually once a day.

POSSIBLE SIDE-EFFECTS MAY INCLUDE: Flushing, dizziness, headache, palpitations, asthenia, rash, chest pain, gastric upset, nausea.

MOTIVAL

POSSIBLE REASONS TO TAKE IT MAY INCLUDE: For the treatment of mixed anxiety/depression.

HOW IS IT PRESCRIBED: Usually three times a day. A course of treatment should be limited to three months.

POSSIBLE SIDE-EFFECTS MAY INCLUDE: Dry mouth, drowsiness, faintness; constipation; increased heart rate, nasal congestion, blurred vision and excitement.

MOTRIN

POSSIBLE REASONS TO TAKE IT MAY INCLUDE: It is usually prescribed for various types of arthritis and soft tissue injuries.

HOW IS IT PRESCRIBED: Usually to be taken as tablets by mouth.

POSSIBLE SIDE-EFFECTS MAY INCLUDE: Nausea, epigastric pain, dizziness, rash, anaemia.

WARNING

You should call your doctor immediately if you develop any side effect while taking a drug. If you do develop side-effects it is vitally important that you speak to your doctor before you stop taking your pills. Remember that this list of side-effects isn't complete – you can develop virtually any side effect with virtually any drug – and remember too that some of these side-effects are quite uncommon and many patients can take a drug without getting any side-effects. Always follow your doctor's advice about how and when to take a drug – and if you are in any doubt at all then ask for a second opinion. The fact that one drug may be accompanied by a long list of possible side-effects does not mean that it is necessarily more or less dangerous or more or less likely to produce problems than a drug which has a shorter list of possible side-effects.

NAPROSYN

POSSIBLE REASONS TO TAKE IT MAY INCLUDE: For the treatment of different types of arthritis.

HOW IS IT PRESCRIBED: Usually once or twice daily.

POSSIBLE SIDE-EFFECTS MAY INCLUDE: Nausea, vomiting, abdominal discomfort, epigastric distress, gastro-intestinal bleeding, peptic ulceration, skin rashes, hair loss, headache, sleeplessness, inability to concentrate, blood problems, tinnitus, hearing impairment, vertigo, jaundice, liver problems, visual disturbances, renal problems.

NAPROXEN

POSSIBLE REASONS TO TAKE IT MAY INCLUDE: For the treatment of different types of arthritis.

HOW IS IT PRESCRIBED: Usually once or twice daily.

POSSIBLE SIDE-EFFECTS MAY INCLUDE: Nausea, vomiting, abdominal discomfort, epigastric distress, gastro-intestinal bleeding, peptic ulceration, skin rashes, hair loss, headache, sleeplessness, inability to concentrate, blood problems, tinnitus, hearing impairment, vertigo, jaundice, liver problems, visual disturbances, kidney problems.

NAVISPARE

POSSIBLE REASONS TO TAKE IT MAY INCLUDE: For the management of mild to moderate hypertension.

HOW IS IT PRESCRIBED: Usually one or two tablets taken once a day in the morning.

POSSIBLE SIDE-EFFECTS MAY INCLUDE: Dizziness, headache, lightheadedness, tiredness, nausea and vomiting, discomfort/pain in the chest, skin rash, loss of appetite, diarrhoea; sleep disturbances, depression; nasal congestion, tinnitus; muscle cramps, joint pain; dryness of mouth, hair loss; blood, heart and liver problems.

WARNING

You should call your doctor immediately if you develop any side effect while taking a drug. If you do develop side-effects it is vitally important that you speak to your doctor before you stop taking your pills. Remember that this list of side-effects isn't complete – you can develop virtually any side effect with virtually any drug – and remember too that some of these side-effects are quite uncommon and many patients can take a drug without getting any side-effects. Always follow your doctor's advice about how and when to take a drug – and if you are in any doubt at all then ask for a second opinion. The fact that one drug may be accompanied by a long list of possible side-effects does not mean that it is necessarily more or less dangerous or more or less likely to produce problems than a drug which has a shorter list of possible side-effects.

NEO-NACLEX

POSSIBLE REASONS TO TAKE IT MAY INCLUDE: Retained fluid, high blood pressure.

HOW IS IT PRESCRIBED: Usually mornings (so that you don't have to pass urine at night).

POSSIBLE SIDE-EFFECTS MAY INCLUDE: Rash, gastrointestinal upset, blood problems, anorexia, dizziness, pancreatitis, impotence.

NIFEDIPINE

POSSIBLE REASONS TO TAKE IT MAY INCLUDE: For the treatment of heart pain and high blood pressure.

HOW IS IT PRESCRIBED: To be taken orally with a little fluid

POSSIBLE SIDE-EFFECTS MAY INCLUDE: Headache, dizziness, flushing, nausea, lethargy, increased frequency of passing urine, dyspepsia, heartburn, palpitation, eye pain, depression.

NIFENSAR XL

POSSIBLE REASONS TO TAKE IT MAY INCLUDE: For the treatment of high blood pressure.

HOW IS IT PRESCRIBED: Usually once a day.

POSSIBLE SIDE-EFFECTS MAY INCLUDE: Headache, dizziness, flushing, rash, nausea, lethargy, tremors, impotence, jaundice.

NITRAZEPAM

POSSIBLE REASONS TO TAKE IT MAY INCLUDE: Nitrazepam is a benzodiazepine with sedative properties. It works in 30 to 60 minutes to produce sleep which lasts for between six and eight hours. The drug is used in the short-term treatment of insomnia when it is severe, disabling or subjecting the individual to unacceptable distress, and where daytime sedation is acceptable.

HOW IS IT PRESCRIBED: To be taken at night. In elderly or debilitated patients dosage should not exceed half doses normally recommended. The dosage should be adjusted on an individual basis. Treatment should, if possible, be intermittent. The lowest dose which can control symptoms should be used and treatment should not be continued at full dose beyond four weeks. Long-term chronic use is not recommended. Treatment should always be tapered off gradually and patients who have taken benzodiazepines for a prolonged time may require a longer period during which doses are reduced. Nitrazepam should not be used alone to treat depression or anxiety associated with depression, since suicide may be precipitated in such patients. In cases of bereavement, psychological adjustment may be inhibited by benzodiazepines. Like all medicaments of this type, nitrazepam may modify patients' performance at skilled tasks (such as driving, operating machinery, etc.) to a varying degree depending upon dosage, administration and individual susceptibility. Alcohol may intensify impairment and should, therefore, be avoided. The dependence potential of the benzodiazepines increases when high doses are used, especially when given over long periods. This is particularly so in patients with a history of alcoholism or drug abuse, or in patients with marked personality disorders. Regular monitoring in such patients is essential. Routine repeat prescriptions should be avoided and treatment should be withdrawn gradually. Symptoms such as depression, nervousness, rebound insomnia, irritability, sweating, and diarrhoea may occur if treatment is suddenly stopped in patients receiving even normal doses for short periods of time. Withdrawal following excessive dosages may produce confusional states, psychotic manifestations and convulsions. An underlying cause for insomnia should be sought before a benzodiazepine is used to treat sleeplessness.

POSSIBLE SIDE-EFFECTS MAY INCLUDE: Drowsiness, sedation, unsteadiness and ataxia; headache, vertigo, hypotension, gastro-intestinal upsets, skin rashes, visual disturbances, changes in libido, urinary retention. Blood dyscrasias, jaundice. Paradoxical aggressive outbursts, excitement, confusion and the uncovering of depression with suicidal tendencies; . The elderly are particularly sensitive to the effects of centrally depressant drugs and may experience confusion, especially if organic brain changes are present. Little is known regarding the efficacy or safety of benzodiazepines in long-term use.

NITROLINGUAL SPRAY

POSSIBLE REASONS TO TAKE IT MAY INCLUDE: For the treatment and prophylaxis of angina pectoris.

HOW IS IT PRESCRIBED: Usually one or two metered doses sprayed under the tongue.

POSSIBLE SIDE-EFFECTS MAY INCLUDE: Headache, postural hypotension, flushing, tachycardia and paradoxical bradycardia, dizziness.

WARNING

You should call your doctor immediately if you develop any side effect while taking a drug. If you do develop side-effects it is vitally important that you speak to your doctor before you stop taking your pills. Remember that this list of side-effects isn't complete – you can develop virtually any side effect with virtually any drug – and remember too that some of these side-effects are quite uncommon and many patients can take a drug without getting any side-effects. Always follow your doctor's advice about how and when to take a drug – and if you are in any doubt at all then ask for a second opinion. The fact that one drug may be accompanied by a long list of possible side-effects does not mean that it is necessarily more or less dangerous or more or less likely to produce problems than a drug which has a shorter list of possible side-effects.

NU-SEALS ASPIRIN

POSSIBLE REASONS TO TAKE IT MAY INCLUDE: Wherever high or prolonged dosage of aspirin is required. It is useful in secondary prophylaxis following myocardial infarction and in patients with unstable angina or cerebral transient ischaemic attacks. Nu-Seals Aspirin is unsuitable for the short-term relief of pain.

HOW IS IT PRESCRIBED: Nu-Seals Aspirin is for oral administration to adults only.

POSSIBLE SIDE-EFFECTS MAY INCLUDE: Hypersensitivity, asthma, urate kidney stones, chronic gastro-intestinal blood loss, tinnitus, nausea and vomiting.

WARNING

You should call your doctor immediately if you develop any side effect while taking a drug. If you do develop side-effects it is vitally important that you speak to your doctor before you stop taking your pills. Remember that this list of side-effects isn't complete – you can develop virtually any side effect with virtually any drug – and remember too that some of these side-effects are quite uncommon and many patients can take a drug without getting any side-effects. Always follow your doctor's advice about how and when to take a drug – and if you are in any doubt at all then ask for a second opinion. The fact that one drug may be accompanied by a long list of possible side-effects does not mean that it is necessarily more or less dangerous or more or less likely to produce problems than a drug which has a shorter list of possible side-effects.

NYCOPREN

POSSIBLE REASONS TO TAKE IT MAY INCLUDE: The treatment of many types of arthritis.

HOW IS IT PRESCRIBED: Usually twice daily.

POSSIBLE SIDE-EFFECTS MAY INCLUDE: Nausea, vomiting, abdominal discomfort, epigastric distress, gastro-intestinal bleeding, peptic ulceration, skin rashes, headache, sleeplessness, inability to concentrate, blood problems, tinnitus, hearing impairment, vertigo, jaundice, liver problems, visual disturbances.

WARNING

You should call your doctor immediately if you develop any side effect while taking a drug. If you do develop side-effects it is vitally important that you speak to your doctor before you stop taking your pills. Remember that this list of side-effects isn't complete – you can develop virtually any side effect with virtually any drug – and remember too that some of these side-effects are quite uncommon and many patients can take a drug without getting any side-effects. Always follow your doctor's advice about how and when to take a drug – and if you are in any doubt at all then ask for a second opinion. The fact that one drug may be accompanied by a long list of possible side-effects does not mean that it is necessarily more or less dangerous or more or less likely to produce problems than a drug which has a shorter list of possible side-effects.

ODRIK

POSSIBLE REASONS TO TAKE IT MAY INCLUDE: For the treatment of high blood pressure.

HOW IS IT PRESCRIBED: Usually once a day.

POSSIBLE SIDE-EFFECTS MAY INCLUDE: Cough, headache, asthenia, dizziness, rash, hypotension, palpitations, angioneurotic oedema.

WARNING

You should call your doctor immediately if you develop any side effect while taking a drug. If you do develop side-effects it is vitally important that you speak to your doctor before you stop taking your pills. Remember that this list of side-effects isn't complete – you can develop virtually any side effect with virtually any drug – and remember too that some of these side-effects are quite uncommon and many patients can take a drug without getting any side-effects. Always follow your doctor's advice about how and when to take a drug – and if you are in any doubt at all then ask for a second opinion. The fact that one drug may be accompanied by a long list of possible side-effects does not mean that it is necessarily more or less dangerous or more or less likely to produce problems than a drug which has a shorter list of possible side-effects.

OMEPRAZOLE

POSSIBLE REASONS TO TAKE IT MAY INCLUDE: For the treatment of oesophageal reflux disease. Treatment of duodenal and benign gastric ulcers.

HOW IS IT PRESCRIBED: Usually once a day.

POSSIBLE SIDE-EFFECTS MAY INCLUDE: skin rash, urticaria and pruritis; photosensitivity, bullous eruption, erythema multiforme, angioedema and alopecia; diarrhoea, headache; constipation, nausea/vomiting, flatulence and abdominal pain; stomatitis and candidiasis; paraesthesia; dizziness, lightheadedness and feeling faint; somnolence, insomnia and vertigo; reversible mental confusion, agitation, depression and hallucinations; arthritic and myalgic symptoms; blurred vision, taste disturbance, peripheral oedema, increased sweating, gynaecomastia, leucopenia, thrombocytopenia, malaise, fever, bronchospasm, encephalopathy in patients with pre-existing severe liver disease, hepatitis with or without jaundice, interstitial nephritis and hepatic failure.

OPTICROM EYE DROPS

POSSIBLE REASONS TO TAKE IT MAY INCLUDE: For the relief and treatment of acute allergic conjunctivitis such as hay fever and chronic allergic conjunctivitis.

HOW IS IT PRESCRIBED: One or two drops into each eye four times daily.

POSSIBLE SIDE-EFFECTS MAY INCLUDE: Transient stinging and burning may occur after instillation.

ORUDIS

POSSIBLE REASONS TO TAKE IT MAY INCLUDE: For the management of rheumatoid arthritis, osteoarthritis, ankylosing spondylitis, acute articular and periarticular disorders, fibrositis, cervical spondylitis, low-back pain, painful musculoskeletal conditions, dysmenorrhoea, acute gout and control of pain and inflammation following orthopaedic surgery.

HOW IS IT PRESCRIBED: Available as capsules and suppositories. Orudis is administered orally and/or rectally; to limit occurrence of gastro-intestinal disturbance, capsules should always be taken with food. Oral dosage is twice daily and should be taken early in the morning and late at night. Rectal dosage is one suppository late at night supplemented as required with the capsules during the daytime.

POSSIBLE SIDE-EFFECTS MAY INCLUDE: Indigestion, dyspepsia, nausea, constipation, diarrhoea, heartburn and various types of abdominal discomfort; headache, dizziness, mild confusion, vertigo, drowsiness, oedema, mood change and insomnia; peptic ulceration, haemorrhage or perforation; thrombocytopenia, hepatic or renal damage, dermatological and photosensitivity reactions, bronchospasm and anaphylaxis.

WARNING
You should call your doctor immediately if you develop any side effect while taking a drug. If you do develop side-effects it is vitally important that you speak to your doctor before you stop taking your pills. Remember that this list of side-effects isn't complete – you can develop virtually any side effect with virtually any drug – and remember too that some of these side-effects are quite uncommon and many patients can take a drug without getting any side-effects. Always follow your doctor's advice about how and when to take a drug – and if you are in any doubt at all then ask for a second opinion. The fact that one drug may be accompanied by a long list of possible side-effects does not mean that it is necessarily more or less dangerous or more or less likely to produce problems than a drug which has a shorter list of possible side-effects.

OXITROPIUM

POSSIBLE REASONS TO TAKE IT MAY INCLUDE: For asthma and similar disorders.

HOW IS IT PRESCRIBED: Usually two or three times a day.

POSSIBLE SIDE-EFFECTS MAY INCLUDE: Blurring of vision, hesitancy of micturition, local irritation of the throat and nose, nausea, dry mouth.

OXIVENT

POSSIBLE REASONS TO TAKE IT MAY INCLUDE: For the treatment of asthma and similar disorders.

HOW IS IT PRESCRIBED: Usually two or three times a day.

POSSIBLE SIDE-EFFECTS MAY INCLUDE: Blurring of vision, hesitancy of micturition, local irritation of the throat and nose, nausea, dry mouth.

OXPRENOLOL

POSSIBLE REASONS TO TAKE IT MAY INCLUDE: For the treatment of high blood pressure, heart pain, heart trouble and anxiety.

HOW IS IT PRESCRIBED: Usually two or three times a day.

POSSIBLE SIDE-EFFECTS MAY INCLUDE: Coldness of hands and feet, hypotension, heart failure; dyspnoea, bronchospasm; skin rash; dizziness, sleep disturbances, headache; nausea, vomiting, flatulence, diarrhoea, constipation, dry mouth; disturbances of vision; loss of libido.

PAVACOL-D

POSSIBLE REASONS TO TAKE IT MAY INCLUDE: For the symptomatic treatment of dry troublesome coughs.

HOW IS IT PRESCRIBED: For adults, usually one or two 5 ml spoonfuls as required. The dosage varies for children according to their age.

POSSIBLE SIDE-EFFECTS MAY INCLUDE: Nausea, drowsiness and constipation. Cough supressants may cause sputum retention which can be harmful in patients with chronic bronchitis and bronchiectasis.

WARNING

You should call your doctor immediately if you develop any side effect while taking a drug. If you do develop side-effects it is vitally important that you speak to your doctor before you stop taking your pills. Remember that this list of side-effects isn't complete – you can develop virtually any side effect with virtually any drug – and remember too that some of these side-effects are quite uncommon and many patients can take a drug without getting any side-effects. Always follow your doctor's advice about how and when to take a drug – and if you are in any doubt at all then ask for a second opinion. The fact that one drug may be accompanied by a long list of possible side-effects does not mean that it is necessarily more or less dangerous or more or less likely to produce problems than a drug which has a shorter list of possible side-effects.

PHYLLOCONTIN CONTINUS

POSSIBLE REASONS TO TAKE IT MAY INCLUDE: For the treatment and prophylaxis of bronchospasm associated with asthma, emphysema and chronic bronchitis. Also indicated in adults for the management of cardiac asthma and left ventricular or congestive cardiac failure.

HOW IS IT PRESCRIBED: Usually every 12 hours; dosage is tailored according to patient's needs.

POSSIBLE SIDE-EFFECTS MAY INCLUDE: Nausea, gastric irritation, headache, palpitations, central nervous system stimulation.

WARNING

You should call your doctor immediately if you develop any side effect while taking a drug. If you do develop side-effects it is vitally important that you speak to your doctor before you stop taking your pills. Remember that this list of side-effects isn't complete – you can develop virtually any side effect with virtually any drug – and remember too that some of these side-effects are quite uncommon and many patients can take a drug without getting any side-effects. Always follow your doctor's advice about how and when to take a drug – and if you are in any doubt at all then ask for a second opinion. The fact that one drug may be accompanied by a long list of possible side-effects does not mean that it is necessarily more or less dangerous or more or less likely to produce problems than a drug which has a shorter list of possible side-effects.

PINDOLOL

POSSIBLE REASONS TO TAKE IT MAY INCLUDE: For the treatment of high blood pressure and angina.

HOW IS IT PRESCRIBED: Usually one, two or three times a day.

POSSIBLE SIDE-EFFECTS MAY INCLUDE: Depression, diarrhoea, nausea, headaches, sleep disturbance, epigastric pain, fatigue, dizziness, low blood pressure, allergic skin reactions, tremors, muscle cramps.

WARNING
You should call your doctor immediately if you develop any side effect while taking a drug. If you do develop side-effects it is vitally important that you speak to your doctor before you stop taking your pills. Remember that this list of side-effects isn't complete – you can develop virtually any side effect with virtually any drug – and remember too that some of these side-effects are quite uncommon and many patients can take a drug without getting any side-effects. Always follow your doctor's advice about how and when to take a drug – and if you are in any doubt at all then ask for a second opinion. The fact that one drug may be accompanied by a long list of possible side-effects does not mean that it is necessarily more or less dangerous or more or less likely to produce problems than a drug which has a shorter list of possible side-effects.

PIROXICAM

POSSIBLE REASONS TO TAKE IT MAY INCLUDE: For a variety of conditions requiring anti-inflammatory and/or analgesic activity, such as rheumatoid arthritis, osteoarthritis, ankylosing spondylitis, acute gout, acute musculoskeletal disorders and juvenile chronic arthritis.

HOW IS IT PRESCRIBED: Available as capsules, dispersible tablets, suppositories and intramuscular injection.

POSSIBLE SIDE-EFFECTS MAY INCLUDE: Stomatitis, anorexia, epigastric distress, nausea, constipation, abdominal discomfort, flatulence, diarrhoea, abdominal pain and indigestion; peptic ulceration, perforation and gastro-intestinal bleeding, in rare cases fatal. Ano-rectal reactions to suppositories have presented as local pain, burning, pruritus, tenesmus. Oedema, mainly of the ankle; possibility of precipitating congestive cardiac failure in elderly patients or those with compromised cardiac function; dizziness, headache, somnolence, insomnia, depression, nervousness, hallucinations, mood alterations, dream abnormalities, mental confusion, paraesthesias and vertigo; rash and pruritus; onycholysis and alopecia; photosensitivity reactions; toxic epidermal necrolysis (Lyell's Disease) and Stevens-Johnson Syndrome; vesiculo-bullous reactions; hypersensitivity reactions such as anaphylaxis, bronchospasm, urticaria/angioneurotic oedema, vasculitis and serum sickness; anaemia, thrombocytopenia, non-thrombocytopenic purpura (Henoch-Schoenlein), leucopenia and eosinophilia; aplastic anaemia, haemolytic anaemia and epistaxis; severe hepatic reactions, including jaundice and cases of fatal hepatitis; palpitations and dyspnoea; metabolic abnormalities such as hypoglycaemia, hyperglycaemia, weight increase or decrease; swollen eyes, blurred vision and eye irritations; malaise, tinnitus.

PLENDIL

POSSIBLE REASONS TO TAKE IT MAY INCLUDE: For the management of high blood pressure.

HOW IS IT PRESCRIBED: Once a day.

POSSIBLE SIDE-EFFECTS MAY INCLUDE: Dizziness, fatigue, headache, ankle swelling, flushing, rash, palpitations, gingival enlargement.

PONSTAN

POSSIBLE REASONS TO TAKE IT MAY INCLUDE: For the management of pain, heavy menstrual bleeding and painful periods.

HOW IS IT PRESCRIBED: Usually three times a day.

POSSIBLE SIDE-EFFECTS MAY INCLUDE: Diarrhoea; skin rash; gastrointestinal bleeding, ulceration and perforation; kidney problems; blood problems; bronchospasm in patients suffering from, or with a previous history of bronchial asthma or allergic disease; liver problems; nausea, vomiting, abdominal pain, headache, facial oedema, anaphylaxis, drowsiness, dizziness.

WARNING
You should call your doctor immediately if you develop any side effect while taking a drug. If you do develop side-effects it is vitally important that you speak to your doctor before you stop taking your pills. Remember that this list of side-effects isn't complete – you can develop virtually any side effect with virtually any drug – and remember too that some of these side-effects are quite uncommon and many patients can take a drug without getting any side-effects. Always follow your doctor's advice about how and when to take a drug – and if you are in any doubt at all then ask for a second opinion. The fact that one drug may be accompanied by a long list of possible side-effects does not mean that it is necessarily more or less dangerous or more or less likely to produce problems than a drug which has a shorter list of possible side-effects.

PREDNESOL TABLETS

POSSIBLE REASONS TO TAKE IT MAY INCLUDE: For the treatment of bronchial asthma, severe hypersensitivity reactions, anaphylaxis; rheumatoid arthritis, systemic lupus erythematosus, dermatomyositis, mixed connective tissue disease (excluding systemic sclerosis), polyarteritis nodosa; inflammatory skin disorders, including pemphigus vulgaris, bullous pemphigoid and pyoderma gangrenosum; minimal change nephrotic syndrome, acute interstitial nephritis; ulcerative colitis, Crohn's disease; sarcoidosis; rheumatic carditis, haemolytic anaemia (autoimmune), acute and lymphatic leukaemia, malignant lymphoma, multiple myeloma, idiopathic thrombocytopenic purpura.

HOW IS IT PRESCRIBED: Varies greatly with condition and individual patient.

POSSIBLE SIDE-EFFECTS MAY INCLUDE: Weight gain, hirsutism, increased appetite; increased susceptibility and severity of infections; osteoporosis, fractures; glaucoma; dyspepsia, peptic ulceration, acute pancreatitis; striae, acne.

PREMPAK-C

POSSIBLE REASONS TO TAKE IT MAY INCLUDE: Menopausal and postmenopausal oestrogen therapy in women with an intact uterus; for sweating and hot flushes; atrophic vaginitis, atrophic urethritis and prophylaxis of osteoporosis in women at risk of developing fractures.

HOW IS IT PRESCRIBED: For maintenance, the lowest effective dose.

POSSIBLE SIDE-EFFECTS MAY INCLUDE: Breakthrough bleeding, spotting, change in menstrual flow, dysmenorrhoea, premenstrual-like syndrome, amenhorrhoea, increase in size of uterine fibromyomata, vaginal candidiasis, change in cervical erosion and in degree of cervical secretion, cystisis-like syndrome; tender breasts, enlarged breasts, breast secretions; nausea, vomiting, abdominal cramps, bloating, cholestatic jaundice; chloasma or melasma which may persist when drug is discontinued, erythema multiforme, erythema nodosum, haemorrhagic eruption, loss of scalp hair, hirsutism; steepening of corneal curvature, intolerance to contact lenses; headaches, migraine, dizziness, mental depression, chorea; increase or decrease in weight, reduced carbohydrate tolerance, aggravation of porphyria, oedema, changes in libido, leg cramps.

PREPULSID

POSSIBLE REASONS TO TAKE IT MAY INCLUDE: For the treatment of dyspepsia, bloating, heartburn, etc.

HOW IS IT PRESCRIBED: Usually three times a day.

POSSIBLE SIDE-EFFECTS MAY INCLUDE: Abdominal cramps, diarrhoea, headaches, lightheadedness.

WARNING

You should call your doctor immediately if you develop any side effect while taking a drug. If you do develop side-effects it is vitally important that you speak to your doctor before you stop taking your pills. Remember that this list of side-effects isn't complete – you can develop virtually any side effect with virtually any drug – and remember too that some of these side-effects are quite uncommon and many patients can take a drug without getting any side-effects. Always follow your doctor's advice about how and when to take a drug – and if you are in any doubt at all then ask for a second opinion. The fact that one drug may be accompanied by a long list of possible side-effects does not mean that it is necessarily more or less dangerous or more or less likely to produce problems than a drug which has a shorter list of possible side-effects.

PRESCAL

POSSIBLE REASONS TO TAKE IT MAY INCLUDE: For the treatment of essential hypertension.

HOW IS IT PRESCRIBED: Usually twice a day.

POSSIBLE SIDE-EFFECTS MAY INCLUDE: Dizziness, flushing, headache, tachycardia, palpitation, weight gain, fatigue, abdominal discomfort, skin rash.

PRIADEL

POSSIBLE REASONS TO TAKE IT MAY INCLUDE: For the treatment of mania, hypomania and some depressions.

HOW IS IT PRESCRIBED: Usually once or twice a day.

POSSIBLE SIDE-EFFECTS MAY INCLUDE: Anorexia, diarrhoea, vomiting, muscle weakness, lack of coordination, drowsiness, lethargy, giddiness, tinnitus, blurred vision, tremor, muscle twitching.

PROCHLORPERAZINE

POSSIBLE REASONS TO TAKE IT MAY INCLUDE: For the treatment of vertigo, nausea, vomiting.

HOW IS IT PRESCRIBED: Usually one, two or three times a day.

POSSIBLE SIDE-EFFECTS MAY INCLUDE: Jaundice, low blood pressure, cardiac arrhythmias, respiratory depression, skin rashes.

PROFLEX CREAM

POSSIBLE REASONS TO TAKE IT MAY INCLUDE: For the treatment of rheumatic and muscular pain, backache, sprains and strains.

HOW IS IT PRESCRIBED: Normally used as cream on the affected area.

POSSIBLE SIDE-EFFECTS MAY INCLUDE: Slight erythema and occasional tingling at the site of application.

PROPRANOLOL

POSSIBLE REASONS TO TAKE IT MAY INCLUDE: For the control of hypertension, the management of angina pectoris; the long-term prophylaxis against reinfarction after recovery from acute myocardial infarction; the control of most forms of cardiac arrythmia; the prophylaxis of migraine; the management of essential tremor, relief of situational anxiety and generalised anxiety symptoms, particularly those of somatic type; prophylaxis of upper gastro-intestinal bleeding in patients with portal hypertension and oesophageal varices; the adjunctive management of thyrotoxicosis and thyrotoxic crisis.

HOW IS IT PRESCRIBED: Usually two, three or four times a day. The dosage depends upon the disorder being treated.

POSSIBLE SIDE-EFFECTS MAY INCLUDE: Bradycardia, heart failure deterioration, postural hypotension which may be associated with syncope, cold extremities; confusion, dizziness, mood changes, nightmares, psychoses and hallucinations, sleep disturbances, hypoglycaemia in children, gastro-intestinal disturbance, purpura, thrombocytopenia, alopecia, dry eyes, psoriasiform skin reactions, exacerbation of psoriasis, skin rashes, paraesthesia; bronchospasm may occur in patients with bronchial asthma or a history of asthmatic complaints, sometimes with fatal outcome; visual disturbances, fatigue and/or lassitude (often transient). Cessation of therapy should be gradual.

WARNING
You should call your doctor immediately if you develop any side effect while taking a drug. If you do develop side-effects it is vitally important that you speak to your doctor before you stop taking your pills. Remember that this list of side-effects isn't complete – you can develop virtually any side effect with virtually any drug – and remember too that some of these side-effects are quite uncommon and many patients can take a drug without getting any side-effects. Always follow your doctor's advice about how and when to take a drug – and if you are in any doubt at all then ask for a second opinion. The fact that one drug may be accompanied by a long list of possible side-effects does not mean that it is necessarily more or less dangerous or more or less likely to produce problems than a drug which has a shorter list of possible side-effects.

PROTHIADEN

POSSIBLE REASONS TO TAKE IT MAY INCLUDE: For the treatment of symptoms of depressive illness, especially where an anti-anxiety effect is required.

HOW IT IS PRESCRIBED: Divided doses or a single dose at night. A daily dose given as a single night-time dose is sometimes more effective and even better tolerated than the conventional divided day-time dosage. There is evidence that this single night-time dose improves the sleep pattern of the depressed patient.

POSSIBLE SIDE-EFFECTS MAY INCLUDE: Atropine-like side-effects including dry mouth, disturbances of accommodation, tachycardia, constipation and hesitancy of micturition; drowsiness, sweating, postural hypotension, tremor and skin rashes; interference with sexual function; depression of the bone marrow, agranulocytosis, hepatitis (including altered liver function), cholestatic jaundice, hypomania and convulsions; psychotic manifestations, including mania and paranoid delusions may be exacerbated during treatment with tricyclic antidepressants. Withdrawal symptoms may occur on abrupt cessation of tricyclic therapy and include insomnia, irritability and excessive perspiration. Similar symptoms in newborn babies whose mothers received tricyclic antidepressants during the third trimester have also been reported. Cardiac arrhythmias and severe hypotension are likely to occur with high dosage or in deliberate overdosage. They may also occur in patients with pre-existing heart disease taking normal dosage. Patients

---

WARNING

You should call your doctor immediately if you develop any side effect while taking a drug. If you do develop side-effects it is vitally important that you speak to your doctor before you stop taking your pills. Remember that this list of side-effects isn't complete – you can develop virtually any side effect with virtually any drug – and remember too that some of these side-effects are quite uncommon and many patients can take a drug without getting any side-effects. Always follow your doctor's advice about how and when to take a drug – and if you are in any doubt at all then ask for a second opinion. The fact that one drug may be accompanied by a long list of possible side-effects does not mean that it is necessarily more or less dangerous than a drug which has a shorter list of possible side-effects.

---

likely to drive vehicles or operate machinery should be warned that the drug may impair alertness. It is recommended that antidepressants should be withdrawn gradually. The elderly are particularly likely to experience adverse reactions to antidepressants, especially agitation, confusion and postural hypotension.

PROZAC

POSSIBLE REASONS TO TAKE IT MAY INCLUDE: Prozac is indicated for the treatment of the symptoms of depressive illness, especially where sedation is not required. It is also used in the treatment of bulimia nervosa.

HOW IS IT PRESCRIBED: For depression in adults a dose of 20 mg/day is recommended. The use of Prozac in children is not recommended, as safety and efficacy have not been established.

POSSIBLE SIDE-EFFECTS MAY INCLUDE: Angioneurotic oedema, urticaria and other allergic reactions; asthenia, fever, nausea, diarrhoea, dry mouth, appetite loss, dyspepsia, vomiting; abnormal liver function tests; headache, nervousness, insomnia, drowsiness, anxiety, tremor, dizziness, fatigue, decreased libido, seizures; hypomania or mania occurred in approximately one per cent of fluoxetine-treated trial patients; dyskinesia, movement disorders developing in patients with risk factors and worsening of pre-existing movement disorders, neuroleptic malignant syndrome-like events; pharyngitis, dyspnoea; pulmonary events, dyspnoea may be the only preceding symptom; rash and/or urticaria; serious systemic reactions, possibly related to vasculitis, have developed in patients with rash, and death has been reported; excessive sweating, serum sickness and anaphylactoid reactions; hair loss, usually reversible; sexual dysfunction (delayed or inhibited orgasm).

WARNING

You should call your doctor immediately if you develop any side effect while taking a drug. If you do develop side-effects it is vitally important that you speak to your doctor before you stop taking your pills. Remember that this list of side-effects isn't complete – you can develop virtually any side effect with virtually any drug – and remember too that some of these side-effects are quite uncommon and many patients can take a drug without getting any side-effects. Always follow your doctor's advice about how and when to take a drug – and if you are in any doubt at all then ask for a second opinion. The fact that one drug may be accompanied by a long list of possible side-effects does not mean that it is necessarily more or less dangerous or more or less likely to produce problems than a drug which has a shorter list of possible side-effects.

RANITIDINE

POSSIBLE REASONS TO TAKE IT MAY INCLUDE: For the treatment of duodenal ulcer and benign gastric ulcer, including that associated with non-steroidal anti-inflammatory agents. In addition, ranitidine is indicated for the prevention of NSAID associated duodenal ulcers. Ranitidine is indicated for the treatment of duodenal ulcers associated with Helicobacter pylori infection and for the treatment of post-operative ulcer, Zollinger-Ellison Syndrome, and oesophageal reflux disease including the long-term management of healed oesophagitis.

HOW IS IT PRESCRIBED: Usually prescribed to be taken twice daily.

POSSIBLE SIDE-EFFECTS MAY INCLUDE: Hepatitis with or without jaundice; acute pancreatitis; leucopenia and thrombocytopenia; agranulocytosis, pancytopenia; hypersensitivity reaction (urticaria, angioneurotic oedema, fever, bronchospasm, hypotension, anaphylactic shock); bradycardia and A-V block; headache, sometimes severe; dizziness; reversible mental confusion, depression and hallucinations, predominantly in severely ill and elderly patients; skin rash, including erythema multiforme; musculoskeletal symptoms such as arthralgia and myalgia; breast symptoms (swelling and/or discomfort) in men.

WARNING

You should call your doctor immediately if you develop any side effect while taking a drug. If you do develop side-effects it is vitally important that you speak to your doctor before you stop taking your pills. Remember that this list of side-effects isn't complete – you can develop virtually any side effect with virtually any drug – and remember too that some of these side-effects are quite uncommon and many patients can take a drug without getting any side-effects. Always follow your doctor's advice about how and when to take a drug – and if you are in any doubt at all then ask for a second opinion. The fact that one drug may be accompanied by a long list of possible side-effects does not mean that it is necessarily more or less dangerous or more or less likely to produce problems than a drug which has a shorter list of possible side-effects.

REGAINE

POSSIBLE REASONS TO TAKE IT MAY INCLUDE: For the treatment of hair loss.

HOW IS IT PRESCRIBED: Usually applied to scalp twice a day.

POSSIBLE SIDE-EFFECTS MAY INCLUDE: Irritant dermatitis, allergic contact dermatitis.

ROHYPNOL

POSSIBLE REASONS TO TAKE IT MAY INCLUDE: Inability to sleep.

HOW IS IT PRESCRIBED: At bedtime. The lowest dose which can control symptoms should be used. Treatment should not be continued at the full dose beyond four weeks. Long-term chronic use is not recommended. Treatment should always be tapered off gradually. Patients who have taken benzodiazepines for a prolonged time may require a longer period during which doses are reduced. Specialist help may be appropriate.

POSSIBLE SIDE-EFFECTS MAY INCLUDE: Drowsiness, confusion, headache, vertigo, hypotension, gastro-intestinal upsets, skin rashes, visual disturbances, changes in libido, urinary retention, blood problems, jaundice. Little is known regarding the efficacy or safety of benzodiazepines in log term use.

SALBULIN

POSSIBLE REASONS TO TAKE IT MAY INCLUDE: For the treatment of asthma.

HOW IS IT PRESCRIBED: Available to be used as an inhaler.

POSSIBLE SIDE-EFFECTS MAY INCLUDE: Mild tremor, headache, increase in heart rate, muscle cramps, palpitations, paradoxical bronchospasm.

SALBUTAMOL

POSSIBLE REASONS TO TAKE IT MAY INCLUDE: For the treatment of asthma.

HOW IS IT PRESCRIBED: Available to be used as tablets, capsules, syrup, inhaler etc.

POSSIBLE SIDE-EFFECTS MAY INCLUDE: Fine muscle tremor, headache, increase in heart rate, muscle cramps, hypersensitivity reactions.

WARNING

You should call your doctor immediately if you develop any side effect while taking a drug. If you do develop side-effects it is vitally important that you speak to your doctor before you stop taking your pills. Remember that this list of side-effects isn't complete – you can develop virtually any side effect with virtually any drug – and remember too that some of these side-effects are quite uncommon and many patients can take a drug without getting any side-effects. Always follow your doctor's advice about how and when to take a drug – and if you are in any doubt at all then ask for a second opinion. The fact that one drug may be accompanied by a long list of possible side-effects does not mean that it is necessarily more or less dangerous or more or less likely to produce problems than a drug which has a shorter list of possible side-effects.

SECURON

POSSIBLE REASONS TO TAKE IT MAY INCLUDE: For the treatment of heart problems and high blood pressure.

HOW IS IT PRESCRIBED: Usually two or three times a day.

POSSIBLE SIDE-EFFECTS MAY INCLUDE: Constipation, flushing, headaches, nausea, vomiting.

SENOKOT

POSSIBLE REASONS TO TAKE IT MAY INCLUDE: For the management of constipation.

HOW IS IT PRESCRIBED: The correct dose is the smallest dose required to produce a comfortable soft-formed motion. It varies between individuals. Senokot is best taken as a single dose, at bedtime by adults and in the morning by children.

POSSIBLE SIDE-EFFECTS MAY INCLUDE: Temporary mild griping during adjustment of dosage.

SEPTRIN

POSSIBLE REASONS TO TAKE IT MAY INCLUDE: For the treatment of infections.

HOW IS IT PRESCRIBED: Usually twice daily.

POSSIBLE SIDE-EFFECTS MAY INCLUDE: Nausea, with or without vomiting; skin rashes; more severe skin sensitivity reactions; blood problems; aseptic meningitis; allergic reactions; shortness of breath, kidney problems; liver problems; diarrhoea, convulsions, vertigo, tinnitus.

SEROPHENE

POSSIBLE REASONS TO TAKE IT MAY INCLUDE: For the treatment of infertility.

HOW IS IT PRESCRIBED: Usually once a day.

POSSIBLE SIDE-EFFECTS MAY INCLUDE: Ovarian enlargement, abdominal/pelvic discomfort, vasomotor symptoms, nausea, vomiting, breast discomfort, visual symptoms, nervousness, insomnia, headache, dizziness, increased urination, heavier periods, depression, fatigue, skin reactions, weight gain, temporary hair loss.

SERTRALINE

POSSIBLE REASONS TO TAKE IT MAY INCLUDE: For the treatment of symptoms of depressive illness.

HOW IS IT PRESCRIBED: Once a day.

POSSIBLE SIDE-EFFECTS MAY INCLUDE: Dry mouth, nausea, diarrhoea, ejaculatory delay, tremor, increased sweating, dyspepsia, insomnia, somnolence.

SIMVASTATIN

POSSIBLE REASONS TO TAKE IT MAY INCLUDE: To lower blood cholesterol.

HOW IS IT PRESCRIBED: Usually once every evening.

POSSIBLE SIDE-EFFECTS MAY INCLUDE: Constipation, flatulence, headache, asthenia, nausea, dyspepsia, abdominal pain, diarrhoea, rash.

SLOW-FE

POSSIBLE REASONS TO TAKE IT MAY INCLUDE: For the prevention and treatment of iron-deficiency anaemia.

HOW IS IT PRESCRIBED: Usually one or two tablets daily.

POSSIBLE SIDE-EFFECTS MAY INCLUDE: Nausea, vomiting, abdominal discomfort, diarrhoea, constipation.

WARNING

You should call your doctor immediately if you develop any side effect while taking a drug. If you do develop side-effects it is vitally important that you speak to your doctor before you stop taking your pills. Remember that this list of side-effects isn't complete – you can develop virtually any side effect with virtually any drug – and remember too that some of these side-effects are quite uncommon and many patients can take a drug without getting any side-effects. Always follow your doctor's advice about how and when to take a drug – and if you are in any doubt at all then ask for a second opinion. The fact that one drug may be accompanied by a long list of possible side-effects does not mean that it is necessarily more or less dangerous or more or less likely to produce problems than a drug which has a shorter list of possible side-effects.

SLOW TRASICOR

POSSIBLE REASONS TO TAKE IT MAY INCLUDE: For the treatment of high blood pressure and angina.

HOW IS IT PRESCRIBED: Usually once a day.

POSSIBLE SIDE-EFFECTS MAY INCLUDE: Dizziness, headache, dry mouth, loss of libido, gastro-intestinal disturbances, low blood pressure, breathing difficulty, heart failure, skin rashes, dry eyes, depression, sleep disturbances.

STEMETIL

POSSIBLE REASONS TO TAKE IT MAY INCLUDE: For the treatment of vertigo, nausea, vomiting.

HOW IS IT PRESCRIBED: Usually one, two or three times a day.

POSSIBLE SIDE-EFFECTS MAY INCLUDE: Jaundice, low blood pressure, cardiac arrhythmias, respiratory depression, skin rashes.

SULINDAC

POSSIBLE REASONS TO TAKE IT MAY INCLUDE: For the treatment of arthritis.

HOW IS IT PRESCRIBED: Usually twice a day.

POSSIBLE SIDE-EFFECTS MAY INCLUDE: Gastro-intestinal pain, dyspepsia, nausea, vomiting, diarrhoea, constipation, flatulence, anorexia, dizziness, headache, nervousness, tinnitus, rash, vertigo, insomnia, sweating, convulsions, depression, psychosis, aseptic meningitis, blood problems, liver problems, kidney problems, heart problems, visual disturbances, decreased hearing, metallic or bitter taste.

WARNING
You should call your doctor immediately if you develop any side effect while taking a drug. If you do develop side-effects it is vitally important that you speak to your doctor before you stop taking your pills. Remember that this list of side-effects isn't complete – you can develop virtually any side effect with virtually any drug – and remember too that some of these side-effects are quite uncommon and many patients can take a drug without getting any side-effects. Always follow your doctor's advice about how and when to take a drug – and if you are in any doubt at all then ask for a second opinion. The fact that one drug may be accompanied by a long list of possible side-effects does not mean that it is necessarily more or less dangerous or more or less likely to produce problems than a drug which has a shorter list of possible side-effects.

SURGAM

POSSIBLE REASONS TO TAKE IT MAY INCLUDE: For the treatment of arthritis, backache, sprains, strains and other pains.

HOW IS IT PRESCRIBED: Usually two or three times a day.

POSSIBLE SIDE-EFFECTS MAY INCLUDE: Dyspepsia, nausea, abdominal pain, vomiting, anorexia, indigestion, heartburn, constipation, gastritis, flatulence, diarrhoea, peptic ulcers, cystitis, headache, drowsiness, skin rash, hair loss.

WARNING

You should call your doctor immediately if you develop any side effect while taking a drug. If you do develop side-effects it is vitally important that you speak to your doctor before you stop taking your pills. Remember that this list of side-effects isn't complete – you can develop virtually any side effect with virtually any drug – and remember too that some of these side-effects are quite uncommon and many patients can take a drug without getting any side-effects. Always follow your doctor's advice about how and when to take a drug – and if you are in any doubt at all then ask for a second opinion. The fact that one drug may be accompanied by a long list of possible side-effects does not mean that it is necessarily more or less dangerous or more or less likely to produce problems than a drug which has a shorter list of possible side-effects.

TAGAMET

POSSIBLE REASONS TO TAKE IT MAY INCLUDE: For the treatment of ulcers in the stomach and duodenum.

HOW IS IT PRESCRIBED: Usually once or twice a day for at least a month.

POSSIBLE SIDE-EFFECTS MAY INCLUDE: Diarrhoea, dizziness, rash, tiredness, swollen breasts in men, liver damage.

TAMOFEN

POSSIBLE REASONS TO TAKE IT MAY INCLUDE: For the management of infertility or breast cancer.

HOW IS IT PRESCRIBED: By mouth.

POSSIBLE SIDE-EFFECTS MAY INCLUDE: Hot flushes, mild nausea, mild thrombocytopenia and leucopenia, pruritis vulvae, skin rash, fluid retention, gastro-intestinal pain; visual disturbance including corneal changes, cataracts and retinopathy; in some pre-menopausal women treated for breast cancer, there is a suppression of menstruation; reversible cystic ovarian swelling has occasionally been observed in this group of patients; endometrial hyperplasia and endometrial polyps; endometrial cancer; abnormal vaginal bleeding, vaginal discharge, pelvic pain or pressure; changes in liver enzyme levels, fatty liver, cholestasis and hepatitis.

TAMOXIFEN

POSSIBLE REASONS TO TAKE IT MAY INCLUDE: For the management of infertility or breast cancer.

HOW IS IT PRESCRIBED: By mouth.

POSSIBLE SIDE-EFFECTS MAY INCLUDE: Hot flushes, mild nausea, mild thrombocytopenia and leucopenia, pruritis vulvae, skin rash, fluid retention, gastro-intestinal pain; visual disturbance including corneal changes, cataracts and retinopathy; in some pre-menopausal women treated for breast cancer, there is a suppression of menstruation; reversible cystic ovarian swelling has occasionally been observed in this group of patients; endometrial hyperplasia and endometrial polyps; endometrial cancer; abnormal vaginal bleeding, vaginal discharge, pelvic pain or pressure; changes in liver enzyme levels, fatty liver, cholestasis and hepatitis.

TEGRETOL

POSSIBLE REASONS TO TAKE IT MAY INCLUDE: For the treatment of epilepsy and the pain of trigeminal neuralgia.

HOW IS IT PRESCRIBED: Usually two or three times a day.

POSSIBLE SIDE-EFFECTS MAY INCLUDE: Dizziness, ataxia, drowsiness, fatigue, headache, blurred vision, depression, hallucinations, appetite loss, agitation, confusion, allergic skin reactions, leucopenia, nausea, vomiting.

TEMAZEPAM

POSSIBLE REASONS TO TAKE IT MAY INCLUDE: Commonly prescribed for the short-term treatment (up to four weeks) of insomnia when it is disabling or subjecting the individual to extreme distress.

HOW IS IT PRESCRIBED: By mouth at night. The lowest dose possible should be used. As with all benzodiazepines, doctors should be aware that long-term use may lead to dependence and withdrawal symptoms in certain patients. Treatment should if possible be intermittent and the drug should not be used for long-term chronic treatment. Elderly patients are likely to respond to smaller doses, possibly half the normal adult dose. All patients taking temazepam should be carefully monitored and routine repeat prescriptions should be avoided. Treatment in all patients should be withdrawn gradually with careful monitoring and reassessment to minimise possible withdrawal symptoms. Patients who have taken benzodiazepines for a long time may require a longer period during which doses are reduced. An underlying cause for insomnia should be sought before deciding on the use of benzodiazepines for symptomatic relief. The risk of dependence increases with higher doses and longer-term use and is further increased in patients with a history of alcoholism, drug abuse or in patients with marked personality disorders. Symptoms such as anxiety, depression, headache, insomnia, tension and sweating have been reported following abrupt discontinuation of benzodiazepines and these symptoms may be difficult to distinguish from the original ones. Other symptoms such as persistent tinnitus, involuntary movements, convulsions and vomiting may be characteristic of benzodiazepine withdrawal syndrome. Patients should be cautioned against driving or operating machinery until it is established that they do not become dizzy or drowsy while taking temazepam. The use of benzodiazepines may release suicidal tendencies in depressed patients.

POSSIBLE SIDE-EFFECTS MAY INCLUDE: Daytime drowsiness, dizziness, muscle weakness, ataxia; amnesia; restlessness, agitation, aggressiveness; blood problems; confusion, depression, fatigue, headache, nausea, sleep disturbance, visual disturbances, gastro intestinal symptoms.

WARNING

You should call your doctor immediately if you develop any side effect while taking a drug. If you do develop side-effects it is vitally important that you speak to your doctor before you stop taking your pills. Remember that this list of side-effects isn't complete – you can develop virtually any side effect with virtually any drug – and remember too that some of these side-effects are quite uncommon and many patients can take a drug without getting any side-effects. Always follow your doctor's advice about how and when to take a drug – and if you are in any doubt at all then ask for a second opinion. The fact that one drug may be accompanied by a long list of possible side-effects does not mean that it is necessarily more or less dangerous or more or less likely to produce problems than a drug which has a shorter list of possible side-effects.

TENORETIC

POSSIBLE REASONS TO TAKE IT MAY INCLUDE: For the management of hypertension.

HOW IS IT PRESCRIBED: Usually one tablet daily.

POSSIBLE SIDE-EFFECTS MAY INCLUDE: Hyperuricaemia, hypokalaemia, impaired glucose tolerance; bradycardia, heart failure deterioration, postural hypotension which may be associated with syncope, cold extremities. Precipitation of heart block, intermittent claudication, Raynaud's phenomenon; confusion, dizziness, headache, mood changes, nightmares, psychoses and hallucinations, sleep disturbances of the type noted with other beta-adrenoceptor blocking drugs; dry mouth, gastro-intestinal disturbances, nausea; leucopenia, purpura, thrombocytopenia; alopecia, dry eyes, psoriasiform skin reactions, exacerbation of psoriasis, skin rashes; paraesthesia; bronchospasm may occur in patients with bronchial asthma or a history of asthmatic complaints; visual disturbances.

WARNING

You should call your doctor immediately if you develop any side effect while taking a drug. If you do develop side-effects it is vitally important that you speak to your doctor before you stop taking your pills. Remember that this list of side-effects isn't complete – you can develop virtually any side effect with virtually any drug – and remember too that some of these side-effects are quite uncommon and many patients can take a drug without getting any side-effects. Always follow your doctor's advice about how and when to take a drug – and if you are in any doubt at all then ask for a second opinion. The fact that one drug may be accompanied by a long list of possible side-effects does not mean that it is necessarily more or less dangerous or more or less likely to produce problems than a drug which has a shorter list of possible side-effects.

TENORMIN

POSSIBLE REASONS TO TAKE IT MAY INCLUDE: For the management of hypertension, angina pectoris, cardiac arrhythmias, myocardial infarction.

HOW IS IT PRESCRIBED: Usually once or twice daily.

POSSIBLE SIDE-EFFECTS MAY INCLUDE: Bradycardia, heart failure deterioration, postural hypotension which may be associated with syncope, cold extremities; precipitation of heart block, intermittent claudication, Raynaud's phenomenon; confusion, dizziness, headache, mood changes, nightmares, psychoses and hallucinations, sleep disturbances of the type noted with other beta-adrenoceptor blocking drugs; dry mouth, gastro-intestinal disturbances; purpura, thrombocytopenia; alopecia, dry eyes, psoriasiform skin reactions, exacerbation of psoriasis, skin rashes; paraesthesia; bronchospasm may occur in patients with bronchial asthma or a history of asthmatic complaints; visual disturbances; fatigue.

WARNING
You should call your doctor immediately if you develop any side effect while taking a drug. If you do develop side-effects it is vitally important that you speak to your doctor before you stop taking your pills. Remember that this list of side-effects isn't complete – you can develop virtually any side effect with virtually any drug – and remember too that some of these side-effects are quite uncommon and many patients can take a drug without getting any side-effects. Always follow your doctor's advice about how and when to take a drug – and if you are in any doubt at all then ask for a second opinion. The fact that one drug may be accompanied by a long list of possible side-effects does not mean that it is necessarily more or less dangerous or more or less likely to produce problems than a drug which has a shorter list of possible side-effects.

TERFENADINE

POSSIBLE REASONS TO TAKE IT MAY INCLUDE: For the relief of hay fever, allergic rhinitis, allergic skin conditions.

HOW IS IT PRESCRIBED: Once or twice a day.

POSSIBLE SIDE-EFFECTS MAY INCLUDE: Abdominal pain, dyspepsia, hair loss and thinning, arrhythmias, confusion, convulsions, depression, dizziness, headache, insomnia, jaundice, liver dysfunction, menstrual disorders, musculoskeletal pain, nightmares, palpitations, skin rash, sweating, tremor, visual disturbances, bronchospasm, anaphylaxis, angioedema.

WARNING

You should call your doctor immediately if you develop any side effect while taking a drug. If you do develop side-effects it is vitally important that you speak to your doctor before you stop taking your pills. Remember that this list of side-effects isn't complete – you can develop virtually any side effect with virtually any drug – and remember too that some of these side-effects are quite uncommon and many patients can take a drug without getting any side-effects. Always follow your doctor's advice about how and when to take a drug – and if you are in any doubt at all then ask for a second opinion. The fact that one drug may be accompanied by a long list of possible side-effects does not mean that it is necessarily more or less dangerous or more or less likely to produce problems than a drug which has a shorter list of possible side-effects.

TERRAMYCIN

POSSIBLE REASONS TO TAKE IT MAY INCLUDE: For the treatment of infections.

HOW IS IT PRESCRIBED: The usual daily dose is 1–2 g, given in four equal doses, depending on the severity of the infection.

POSSIBLE SIDE-EFFECTS MAY INCLUDE: Anorexia, nausea, vomiting, diarrhoea, glossitis, dysphagia, enterocolitis, and inflammatory lesions (with candidial overgrowth) in the anogenital regions. Oesophagitis and oesophageal ulceration; maculopapular and erythematous rashes; exfoliative dermatitis; photosensitvity manifested by an exaggerated sunburn reaction; urticaria, angioneurotic oedema, anaphylaxis, anaphylactoid purpura, pericarditis, and exacerbation of systemic lupus erythematosus; bulging fontanellas in infants and benign intracranial hypertension in adults; haemolytic anaemia, thrombocytopenia, neutropenia and eosinophilia.

WARNING

You should call your doctor immediately if you develop any side effect while taking a drug. If you do develop side-effects it is vitally important that you speak to your doctor before you stop taking your pills. Remember that this list of side-effects isn't complete – you can develop virtually any side effect with virtually any drug – and remember too that some of these side-effects are quite uncommon and many patients can take a drug without getting any side-effects. Always follow your doctor's advice about how and when to take a drug – and if you are in any doubt at all then ask for a second opinion. The fact that one drug may be accompanied by a long list of possible side-effects does not mean that it is necessarily more or less dangerous or more or less likely to produce problems than a drug which has a shorter list of possible side-effects.

THYROXINE

POSSIBLE REASONS TO TAKE IT MAY INCLUDE: For the treatment of hypothyroidism.

HOW IS IT PRESCRIBED: Dosage tailored for each patient's needs.

POSSIBLE SIDE-EFFECTS MAY INCLUDE: Anginal pain, cardiac arrhythmias, palpitation, and cramps in skeletal muscle; also tachycardia, diarrhoea, vomiting, tremors, restlessness, excitability, insomnia, headache, flushing, sweating, excessive loss of weight and muscular weakness.

TIAPROFENIC ACID

POSSIBLE REASONS TO TAKE IT MAY INCLUDE: For the treatment of arthritis, backache, sprains, strains and other pains.

HOW IS IT PRESCRIBED: Usually two or three times a day.

POSSIBLE SIDE-EFFECTS MAY INCLUDE: Dyspepsia, nausea, abdominal pain, vomiting, anorexia, indigestion, heartburn, constipation, gastritis, flatulence, diarrhoea, peptic ulcers, cystitis, headache, drowsiness, skin rash, hair loss.

WARNING

You should call your doctor immediately if you develop any side effect while taking a drug. If you do develop side-effects it is vitally important that you speak to your doctor before you stop taking your pills. Remember that this list of side-effects isn't complete – you can develop virtually any side effect with virtually any drug – and remember too that some of these side-effects are quite uncommon and many patients can take a drug without getting any side-effects. Always follow your doctor's advice about how and when to take a drug – and if you are in any doubt at all then ask for a second opinion. The fact that one drug may be accompanied by a long list of possible side-effects does not mean that it is necessarily more or less dangerous or more or less likely to produce problems than a drug which has a shorter list of possible side-effects.

TILDIEM

POSSIBLE REASONS TO TAKE IT MAY INCLUDE: For the management of angina pectoris.

HOW IS IT PRESCRIBED: Usually three times a day.

POSSIBLE SIDE-EFFECTS MAY INCLUDE: Ankle oedema, malaise, headache, hot flushes, gastrointestinal disturbances.

TIMOLOL

POSSIBLE REASONS TO TAKE IT MAY INCLUDE: For the treatment of high blood pressure, heart disease and migraine.

HOW IS IT PRESCRIBED: Usually once or twice a day.

POSSIBLE SIDE-EFFECTS MAY INCLUDE: Fatigue, weakness, heart failure, coldness of limb extremities, low blood pressure, heart block, epigastric distress, nausea, vomiting, dizziness, disorientation, vertigo, paraesthesia, headache, hallucinations, nightmares, insomnia, depression, breathing difficulty, skin rashes, dry eyes.

WARNING

You should call your doctor immediately if you develop any side effect while taking a drug. If you do develop side-effects it is vitally important that you speak to your doctor before you stop taking your pills. Remember that this list of side-effects isn't complete – you can develop virtually any side effect with virtually any drug – and remember too that some of these side-effects are quite uncommon and many patients can take a drug without getting any side-effects. Always follow your doctor's advice about how and when to take a drug – and if you are in any doubt at all then ask for a second opinion. The fact that one drug may be accompanied by a long list of possible side-effects does not mean that it is necessarily more or less dangerous or more or less likely to produce problems than a drug which has a shorter list of possible side-effects.

TRANDATE

POSSIBLE REASONS TO TAKE IT MAY INCLUDE: For the treatment of high blood pressure and heart pain.

HOW IS IT PRESCRIBED: Usually twice a day.

POSSIBLE SIDE-EFFECTS MAY INCLUDE: Headache, tiredness, dizziness, depressed mood, lethargy, nasal congestion, sweating, ankle swelling, tingling sensation in the scalp, acute retention of urine, difficulty in passing urine, ejaculatory failure, epigastric pain, nausea, vomiting, rash, itching, difficulty in breathing, heart block and jaundice.

TRANDOLAPRIL

POSSIBLE REASONS TO TAKE IT MAY INCLUDE: For the treatment of high blood pressure.

HOW IS IT PRESCRIBED: Usually once a day.

POSSIBLE SIDE-EFFECTS MAY INCLUDE: Cough, headache, asthenia, dizziness, rash, hypotension, palpitations, angioneurotic oedema, nausea.

TRASICOR

POSSIBLE REASONS TO TAKE IT MAY INCLUDE: For the treatment of high blood pressure, heart pain, heart trouble and anxiety.

HOW IS IT PRESCRIBED: Usually two or three times a day.

POSSIBLE SIDE-EFFECTS MAY INCLUDE: Coldness of hands and feet, hypotension, heart failure; dyspnoea, bronchospasm; skin rash; dizziness, sleep disturbances, headache; nausea, vomiting, flatulence, diarrhoea, constipation, dry mouth; disturbances of vision; loss of libido.

TRILUDAN

POSSIBLE REASONS TO TAKE IT MAY INCLUDE: For the relief of hay fever, allergic rhinitis, allergic skin conditions.

HOW IS IT PRESCRIBED: Once or twice a day.

POSSIBLE SIDE-EFFECTS MAY INCLUDE: Abdominal pain, dyspepsia, hair loss and thinning, arrhythmias, confusion, convulsions, depression, dizziness, headache, insomnia, jaundice, liver dysfunction, menstrual disorders, musculoskeletal pain, nightmares, palpitations, skin rash, sweating, tremor, visual disturbances, bronchospasm, anaphylaxis, angioedema.

WARNING

You should call your doctor immediately if you develop any side effect while taking a drug. If you do develop side-effects it is vitally important that you speak to your doctor before you stop taking your pills. Remember that this list of side-effects isn't complete – you can develop virtually any side effect with virtually any drug – and remember too that some of these side-effects are quite uncommon and many patients can take a drug without getting any side-effects. Always follow your doctor's advice about how and when to take a drug – and if you are in any doubt at all then ask for a second opinion. The fact that one drug may be accompanied by a long list of possible side-effects does not mean that it is necessarily more or less dangerous or more or less likely to produce problems than a drug which has a shorter list of possible side-effects.

TYLEX

POSSIBLE REASONS TO TAKE IT MAY INCLUDE: For the relief of severe pain.

HOW IS IT PRESCRIBED: Usually one to two capsules every four hours as required.

POSSIBLE SIDE-EFFECTS MAY INCLUDE: Lightheadedness, dizziness, sedation, shortness of breath, nausea and vomiting. These effects seem more prominent in ambulatory than non-ambulatory patients and some of these adverse reactions may be alleviated if the patient lies down. Other adverse reactions include allergic reactions, euphoria, dysphoria, constipation, abdominal pain and pruritis.

VALIUM ROCHE

POSSIBLE REASONS TO TAKE IT MAY INCLUDE: Commonly used in the short-term (two to four weeks) symptomatic treatment of anxiety that is severe, disabling or subjecting the individual to unacceptable distress, occurring alone or in association with insomnia or short-term psychosomatic, organic or psychotic illness. Also for short-term (two to four weeks) treatment of conditions where anxiety may be a precipitating or aggravating factor, e.g. tension headaches or migraine attacks.

HOW IS IT PRESCRIBED: The usual dose is 2 mg three times daily. The maximum dose is up to 30 mg daily in divided doses. For insomnia associated with anxiety 5–15 mg before retiring. The lowest dose which can control symptoms should be used. Treatment should not be continued at the full dose beyond four weeks. Long-term chronic use is not recommended. Treatment should always be tapered off gradually. Patients who have taken benzodiazepines for a prolonged time may require a longer period during which doses are reduced. Specialist help may be appropriate. When given to elderly or debilitated patients, doses should not exceed half those normally recommended.

POSSIBLE SIDE-EFFECTS MAY INCLUDE: Like all medicaments of this type, Valium Roche may modify patients' performance at skilled tasks (driving, operating machinery, etc.) to a varying degree depending on dosage, administration and individual susceptibility. Alcohol may intensify any impairment and should, therefore, be avoided during treat-

---

WARNING

You should call your doctor immediately if you develop any side effect while taking a drug. If you do develop side-effects it is vitally important that you speak to your doctor before you stop taking your pills. Remember that this list of side-effects isn't complete – you can develop virtually any side effect with virtually any drug – and remember too that some of these side-effects are quite uncommon and many patients can take a drug without getting any side-effects. Always follow your doctor's advice about how and when to take a drug – and if you are in any doubt at all then ask for a second opinion. The fact that one drug may be accompanied by a long list of possible side-effects does not mean that it is necessarily more or less dangerous or more or less likely to produce problems than a drug which has a shorter list of possible side-effects.

---

ment. Valium Roche should not be used alone to treat depression or anxiety associated with depression, since suicide may be precipitated in such patients. Amnesia may occur. In cases of bereavement, psychological adjustments may be inhibited by benzodiazepines. The dependence potential of the benzodiazepines increases when high doses are used, especially when given over long periods. This is particularly so in patients with a history of alcoholism or drug abuse or in patients with marked personality disorders. Treatment should be withdrawn gradually. Symptoms such as depression, nervousness, rebound insomnia, irritability, sweating, and diarrhoea have been reported following abrupt cessation of treatment in patients receiving even normal therapeutic doses for short periods of time. Withdrawal following excessive dosages may produce confusional states, psychotic manifestations and convulsions. Abnormal psychological reactions to benzodiazepines have been reported. Behavioural effects include paradoxical aggressive outbursts, excitement, confusion, and the uncovering of depression with suicidal tendencies. Extreme caution should therefore be used in prescribing benzodiazepines to patients with personality disorders. In patients with myasthenia gravis, who are prescribed Valium Roche, care should be taken on account of pre-existing muscle weakness. Common adverse effects include drowsiness, sedation, unsteadiness and ataxia, these are dose related and may persist into the following day, even after a single dose. Other adverse effects include headache, vertigo, hypotension, gastro-intestinal upsets, skin rashes, visual disturbances, changes in libido, urinary retention, blood dyscrasias and jaundice. Little is known regarding the efficacy or safety of benzodiazepines in long-term use.

WARNING

You should call your doctor immediately if you develop any side effect while taking a drug. If you do develop side-effects it is vitally important that you speak to your doctor before you stop taking your pills. Remember that this list of side-effects isn't complete – you can develop virtually any side effect with virtually any drug – and remember too that some of these side-effects are quite uncommon and many patients can take a drug without getting any side-effects. Always follow your doctor's advice about how and when to take a drug – and if you are in any doubt at all then ask for a second opinion. The fact that one drug may be accompanied by a long list of possible side-effects does not mean that it is necessarily more or less dangerous or more or less likely to produce problems than a drug which has a shorter list of possible side-effects.

VENTOLIN

POSSIBLE REASONS TO TAKE IT MAY INCLUDE: For the treatment of asthma.

HOW IS IT PRESCRIBED: Available to be used as tablets, capsules, syrup, inhaler etc

POSSIBLE SIDE-EFFECTS MAY INCLUDE: Fine muscle tremor, headache, increase in heart rate, muscle cramps, hypersensitivity reactions.

WARNING

You should call your doctor immediately if you develop any side effect while taking a drug. If you do develop side-effects it is vitally important that you speak to your doctor before you stop taking your pills. Remember that this list of side-effects isn't complete – you can develop virtually any side effect with virtually any drug – and remember too that some of these side-effects are quite uncommon and many patients can take a drug without getting any side-effects. Always follow your doctor's advice about how and when to take a drug – and if you are in any doubt at all then ask for a second opinion. The fact that one drug may be accompanied by a long list of possible side-effects does not mean that it is necessarily more or less dangerous or more or less likely to produce problems than a drug which has a shorter list of possible side-effects.

VERAPAMIL

POSSIBLE REASONS TO TAKE IT MAY INCLUDE: For the treatment of heart problems and high blood pressure.

HOW IS IT PRESCRIBED: Usually two or three times a day.

POSSIBLE SIDE-EFFECTS MAY INCLUDE: Constipation, flushing, headaches, nausea, vomiting.

VISKEN

POSSIBLE REASONS TO TAKE IT MAY INCLUDE: For the treatment of high blood pressure and angina.

HOW IS IT PRESCRIBED: Usually one, two or three times a day.

POSSIBLE SIDE-EFFECTS MAY INCLUDE: Depression, diarrhoea, nausea, headaches, sleep disturbance, epigastric pain, fatigue, dizziness, low blood pressure, allergic skin reactions, muscle cramps, tremors.

VOLTAROL

POSSIBLE REASONS TO TAKE IT MAY INCLUDE: For the relief of all grades of pain and inflammation in a wide range of conditions, including: arthritic conditions: rheumatoid arthritis, osteoarthritis, ankylosing spondylitis, acute gout; acute musculoskeletal disorders such as periarthritis (e.g. frozen shoulder), tendinitis, tenosynovitis, bursitis; other painful conditions resulting from trauma, including fracture, low back pain, sprains, strains, dislocations, orthopaedic, dental and other minor surgery.

HOW IS IT PRESCRIBED: More suitable for short-term use in acute conditions for which treatment is required for no more than three months. There is no information on the use of Voltarol for more than three months. Usually taken two or three times a day.

POSSIBLE SIDE-EFFECTS MAY INCLUDE: epigastric pain, other gastro-intestinal disorders (e.g. nausea, vomiting, diarrhoea, abdominal cramps, dyspepsia, flatulence, anorexia); gastro-intestinal bleeding, peptic ulcer (with or without bleeding or perforation), bloody diarrhoea; lower-gut disorders (e.g. non-specific haemorrhagic colitis and exacerbations of ulcerative colitis or crohn's proctocolitis), pancreatitis, aphthous stomatitis, glossitis, oesophageal lesions, constipation; headache, dizziness, or vertigo; drowsiness, tiredness; disturbances of sensation, paraesthesia, memory disturbance, disorientation, disturbance of vision (blurred vision, diplopia), impaired hearing, tinnitus, insomnia,

---

WARNING

You should call your doctor immediately if you develop any side effect while taking a drug. If you do develop side-effects it is vitally important that you speak to your doctor before you stop taking your pills. Remember that this list of side-effects isn't complete – you can develop virtually any side effect with virtually any drug – and remember too that some of these side-effects are quite uncommon and many patients can take a drug without getting any side-effects. Always follow your doctor's advice about how and when to take a drug – and if you are in any doubt at all then ask for a second opinion. The fact that one drug may be accompanied by a long list of possible side-effects does not mean that it is necessarily more or less dangerous or more or less likely to produce problems than a drug which has a shorter list of possible side-effects.

---

irritability, convulsions, depression, anxiety, nightmares, tremor, psychotic reactions. Taste alteration disorders; rashes or skin eruptions, urticaria; bullous eruptions, eczema, erythema multiforme, Stevens-Johnson Syndrome, Lyell's Syndrome, (acute toxic epidermolysis), erythroderma (exfoliative dermatitis), loss of hair, photosensitivity reactions, purpura including allergic purpura; acute renal insufficiency, urinary abnormalities (e.g. haematuria, proteinuria), interstitial nephritis, nephrotic syndrome, papillary necrosis; liver problems including hepatitis (in isolated cases fulminant) with or without jaundice; thrombocytopenia, leucopenia, agranulocytosis, haemolytic anaemia, aplastic anaemia; oedema, hypersensitivity reactions (e.g. bronchospasm, anaphylactic/anaphylactoid systemic reactions including hypotension); impotence, palpitation, chest pain, hypertension.

ZANTAC

POSSIBLE REASONS TO TAKE IT MAY INCLUDE: For the treatment of duodenal ulcer and benign gastric ulcer, including that associated with non-steroidal anti-inflammatory agents. In addition, Zantac tablets and syrup are indicated for the prevention of NSAID associated duodenal ulcers. Zantac tablets are indicated for the treatment of duodenal ulcers associated with Helicobacter pylori infection. Zantac tablets and syrup are also indicated for the treatment of post-operative ulcer, Zollinger-Ellison Syndrome, and oesophageal reflux disease including the long-term management of healed oesophagitis.

HOW IS IT PRESCRIBED: Usually prescribed to be taken twice daily.

POSSIBLE SIDE-EFFECTS MAY INCLUDE: Hepatitis with or without jaundice; acute pancreatitis; leucopenia and thrombocytopenia; agranulocytosis, pancytopenia; hypersensitivity reaction (urticaria, angioneurotic oedema, fever, bronchospasm, hypotension, anaphylactic shock); bradycardia and A-V block; headache, sometimes severe; dizziness; reversible mental confusion, depression and hallucinations, predominantly in severely ill and elderly patients; skin rash, including erythema multiforme; musculoskeletal symptoms such as arthralgia and myalgia; breast symptoms (swelling and/or discomfort) in men.

WARNING
You should call your doctor immediately if you develop any side effect while taking a drug. If you do develop side-effects it is vitally important that you speak to your doctor before you stop taking your pills. Remember that this list of side-effects isn't complete – you can develop virtually any side effect with virtually any drug – and remember too that some of these side-effects are quite uncommon and many patients can take a drug without getting any side-effects. Always follow your doctor's advice about how and when to take a drug – and if you are in any doubt at all then ask for a second opinion. The fact that one drug may be accompanied by a long list of possible side-effects does not mean that it is necessarily more or less dangerous or more or less likely to produce problems than a drug which has a shorter list of possible side-effects.

ZESTRIL

POSSIBLE REASONS TO TAKE IT MAY INCLUDE: For the treatment of high blood pressure (hypertension) and heart failure.

HOW IS IT PRESCRIBED: Usually once a day; the dosage depends upon the patient's condition and symptoms.

POSSIBLE SIDE-EFFECTS MAY INCLUDE: Hypotension; angioneurotic oedema of the face, extremities, lips, tongue, glottis and/ or larynx; dizziness, headache, diarrhoea, fatigue, cough and nausea; rash, and asthenia; myocardial infarction or cerebrovascular accident possibly secondary to excessive hypotension in high-risk patients, palpitation, tachycardia, pancreatitis, abdominal pain, dry mouth, hepatitis (hepatocellular or cholestatic), mood alterations, mental confusion, urticaria, diaphoresis, uraemia, oliguria/anuria, renal dysfunction, acute renal failure, impotence; haemolytic anaemia; symptom complex which may include fever, vasculitis, myalgia arthralgia/arthritis, a positive ANA, elevated erythrocyte sedimentation rate, eosinophilia, and leucocytosis; photosensitivity.

WARNING

You should call your doctor immediately if you develop any side effect while taking a drug. If you do develop side-effects it is vitally important that you speak to your doctor before you stop taking your pills. Remember that this list of side-effects isn't complete – you can develop virtually any side effect with virtually any drug – and remember too that some of these side-effects are quite uncommon and many patients can take a drug without getting any side-effects. Always follow your doctor's advice about how and when to take a drug – and if you are in any doubt at all then ask for a second opinion. The fact that one drug may be accompanied by a long list of possible side-effects does not mean that it is necessarily more or less dangerous or more or less likely to produce problems than a drug which has a shorter list of possible side-effects.

ZOCOR

POSSIBLE REASONS TO TAKE IT MAY INCLUDE: To lower blood cholesterol.

HOW IS IT PRESCRIBED: Usually once every evening.

POSSIBLE SIDE-EFFECTS MAY INCLUDE: Constipation, flatulence, headache, asthenia, nausea, dyspepsia, abdominal pain, diarrhoea, rash.

ZOVIRAX TABLETS

POSSIBLE REASONS TO TAKE IT MAY INCLUDE: For the treatment of herpes simplex virus infections of the skin and mucous membranes including initial and recurrent genital herpes.

HOW IS IT PRESCRIBED: Tablets should usually be taken five times daily at approximately four-hourly intervals omitting the night-time dose. Treatment should continue for five days, but in severe initial infections this may have to be extended.

POSSIBLE SIDE-EFFECTS MAY INCLUDE: Skin rashes; gastrointestinal effects including nausea, vomiting, diarrhoea and abdominal pains; reversible neurological reactions, notably dizziness, confusional states, hallucinations and somnolence; accelerated diffuse hair loss; mild, transient rises in bilirubin and liver-related enzymes, small increases in blood urea and creatinine, small decreases in haemotological indices; headaches.

ZYLORIC

POSSIBLE REASONS TO TAKE IT MAY INCLUDE: For the treatment of gout and renal stones.

HOW IS IT PRESCRIBED: The dosage is adjusted by monitoring serum urate concentrations and urinary urate/uric acid levels.

POSSIBLE SIDE-EFFECTS MAY INCLUDE: Skin reactions may be pruritic, maculopapular, sometimes scaly, sometimes purpuric and rarely exfoliative; fever, lymphadenopathy, arthralgia and/or eosinophilia resembling Stevens-Johnson and/or Lyell Syndrome; hepatitis, interstitial nephritis, epilepsy; angioimmunoblastic lymphadenopathy; granulomatous hepatitis, without overt evidence of more generalised hypersensitivity; nausea and vomiting; recurrent haematemesis, steatorrhoea; thrombocytopenia, agranulocytosis and aplastic anaemia; fever, general malaise, asthenia, headache, vertigo, ataxia, somnolence, coma, depression, paralysis, paraesthesiae, neuropathy, visual disorder, cataract, macular changes, taste perversion, stomatitis, changed bowel habit, infertility, impotence, nocturnal emission, diabetes mellitus, hyperlipaemia, furunculosis, alopecia, discoloured hair, angina, hypertension, bradycardia, oedema, uraemia, haematuria, gynaecomastia.

WARNING

You should call your doctor immediately if you develop any side effect while taking a drug. If you do develop side-effects it is vitally important that you speak to your doctor before you stop taking your pills. Remember that this list of side-effects isn't complete – you can develop virtually any side effect with virtually any drug – and remember too that some of these side-effects are quite uncommon and many patients can take a drug without getting any side-effects. Always follow your doctor's advice about how and when to take a drug – and if you are in any doubt at all then ask for a second opinion. The fact that one drug may be accompanied by a long list of possible side-effects does not mean that it is necessarily more or less dangerous or more or less likely to produce problems than a drug which has a shorter list of possible side-effects.

Also available by Vernon Coleman

How To Overcome Toxic Stress
and the Twentieth Century Blues

*'Never have I read a book that is so startlingly true. I was
dumbfounded by your wisdom. You will go down in history as one of
the truly great health reformers of our time'*
(Extracted from a letter to the author)

If you are frustrated, bored, lonely, angry, sad, tired, listless, frightened,
unhappy or tearful then it is possible that you are suffering from Toxic
Stress.

After two decades of research Dr Coleman has come up with his
own antidote to Toxic Stress which he shares with you in this inspira-
tional book. In order to feel well and happy again you need to take a close
look at your life and put things back in the right order. Dr Coleman shows
you how to value the worthwhile things in life and give less time to
things which matter very little at all. The book contains hundreds of practical tips on how to cope with the stresses and strains of daily life.

*"This book is absolutely outstanding because it addresses a serious
problem which up until now has not been identified or discussed in any
meaningful way. If you feel you have a lot of stress being generated
from outside your life, this book is an absolute must. Personally, I am
going to get five copies so that I can put them in my lending library
and lend them to as many people as I can"*
(Health Consciousness, USA)

Price £9.95

Published by EMJ Books
Order from Publishing House, Trinity Place, Barnstaple,
Devon EX32 9HJ, England

Also available by Vernon Coleman

Bodypower
The secret of self-healing

A new edition of the sensational book which hit the Sunday Times bestseller list and the Bookseller Top Ten Chart.

This international bestseller shows you how you can harness your body's amazing powers to help you cure 9 out of 10 illnesses without seeing a doctor!

The book also covers:

- How your personality affects your health
- How to stay slim for life
- How to improve your eyesight
- How to break bad habits
- How to relax your body and mind
- How to improve your figure
- And much much more!

"Don't miss it. Dr Coleman's theories could change your life"
(Sunday Mirror)

"A marvellously succinct and simple account of how the body can heal itself without resort to drugs"
(The Spectator)

"Could make stress a thing of the past"
(Woman's World)

Price £9.95

Published by EMJ Books
Order from Publishing House, Trinity Place, Barnstaple, Devon EX32 9HJ, England

Also available by Vernon Coleman

Mindpower

Nothing has the potential to influence your health quite as much as your mind. We've all heard the phrase "you'll worry yourself to death" and scientists have now proved that it is indeed possible for your mind to at least make you ill if not actually kill you. Most doctors around the world now agree that at least 75% of all illnesses can be caused or made worse by stress and/or anxiety. But although your mind can make you ill it can also make you better and has an enormous capacity to heal and cure if only you know how to harness its extraordinary powers and make them work for you - instead of against you!

You can use Mindpower to help you deal with a range of problems including: Anxiety, Depression, Arthritis, Cancer, Asthma, Diabetes, Eczema, Headaches, Heart Disease, High Blood Pressure, Indigestion, Women's Problems, Migraine, Pain, Sleeplessness.

"Dr Coleman's Mindpower is based on an inspiring message of hope."
(Western Morning News)

"... offers an insight into the most powerful healing agent in the world - the power of the mind."
(Birmingham Post)

"Dr. Coleman explains the importance of a patient's mental attitude in controlling and treating illness, and suggests some easy to learn techniques."
(Woman's World)

"I thoroughly enjoyed it and am sure it will be another bestseller."
(Nursing Times)

Price £9.95

Published by EMJ Books
Order from Publishing House, Trinity Place, Barnstaple,
Devon EX32 9HJ, England

Also available by Vernon Coleman

Betrayal of Trust

Vernon Coleman catalogues the incompetence and dishonesty of the medical profession and the pharmaceutical industry and explains the historical background to the problems which exist today in the world of healthcare. He shows how drugs are put onto the market without being properly tested, and provides hard evidence for his astonishing assertion that doctors do more harm than good.

"I found (it) so brilliant I could not stop reading it"
(A.P., Luton)

"I urge anyone interested in medicine and the safety of drugs to read Betrayal of Trust"
(Leicester Mercury)

"I feel you should be congratulated for producing something that should be required reading for both consumers and producers of the health service"
(R.P., Senior Lecturer in Psychology)

"Only 15% of medical interventions are supported by solid scientific evidence ... one in six hospital patients are there because of doctor-induced disease ... only 1% of medical articles in medical journals are scientifically sound. The ingredients for this further blast against the medical establishment from bestselling doctor-author Vernon Coleman certainly make for a rattling good read"
(The Good Book Guide)

Price £9.95

Published by EMJ Books
Order from Publishing House, Trinity Place, Barnstaple,
Devon EX32 9HJ, England

Also available by Vernon Coleman

Food For Thought

In this bestselling book Dr Coleman explains which foods to avoid and which to eat to reduce your risk of developing cancer. He also lists foods known to be associated with a wide range of other diseases including Asthma, Gall Bladder Disease, Headaches , Heart Trouble, High Blood Pressure, Indigestion and many more.

Years of research have gone into the writing of this book which explains the facts about mad cow disease, vegetarian eating, microwaves, drinking water, food poisoning, food irradiation and additives. It contains all the information you need about vitamins, carbohydrates, fats and proteins plus a list of 20 superfoods which Dr Coleman believes can improve your health and protect you from a wide range of health problems. The book also includes a "slim-for-life" programme with 48 quick slimming tips to help you lose weight safely and permanently.

" ... a guide to healthy eating which reads like a thriller.. advice on vitamins, minerals, healthy drinking, losing weight and much more. If you're worried about what you eat, this will tell you what to avoid"
(The Good Book Guide)

" .. his no nonsense approach to all foods makes finding your way through the nutritional maze that much easier"
(Evening Times)

"I consider it to be one of the most brilliant books of its kind that I have ever read. Not only are the contents a mine of information and advice but the style is such that it makes the whole so thoroughly enjoyable to read; indeed it is a book difficult to put down"
(G.P. Stretham)

Price £9.95
Published by EMJ Books
Order from Publishing House, Trinity Place, Barnstaple,
Devon EX32 9HJ, England